Cherokee Medicine, Colonial Germs

New Directions in Native American Studies
Colin G. Calloway and K. Tsianina Lomawaima, General Editors

CHEROKEE MEDICINE, COLONIAL GERMS

An Indigenous Nation's
Fight against Smallpox, 1518–1824

Paul Kelton

UNIVERSITY OF OKLAHOMA PRESS : NORMAN

Library of Congress Cataloging-in-Publication Data

Kelton, Paul, author.
  Cherokee medicine, colonial germs : an indigenous nation's fight against
smallpox, 1518–1824 / Paul Kelton.
      p. ; cm.
  Includes bibliographical references and index.
  ISBN 978-0-8061-4688-1 (hardcover : alk. paper)
  I. Title
  [DNLM: 1. Indians, North American—history—Southeastern United States.
2. Smallpox—history—Southeastern United States. 3. Colonialism—history—
Southeastern United States. 4. History, 16th Century—Southeastern United
States. 5. History, Modern 1601—Southeastern United States. 6. Smallpox
Vaccine—history—Southeastern United States. WC 585]
  RA644.S6
  614.5'20975—dc23
                                                                2014030514

*Cherokee Medicine, Colonial Germs: An Indigenous Nation's Fight against Smallpox,
1518–1824* is Volume 11 in the New Directions in Native American Studies series.

The paper in this book meets the guidelines for permanence and durability of
the Committee on Production Guidelines for Book Longevity of the Council
on Library Resources, Inc. ∞

2 3 4 5 6 7 8 9 10

For Stephanie

CONTENTS

Illustrations

Figures

Maps

ACKNOWLEDGMENTS

Without the support of numerous individuals and institutions, this project would not have been possible. I have relied heavily on the Interlibrary Loan Staff at the University of Kansas for assistance tracking down and acquiring hard to find materials, and I especially appreciate the generous assistance of Nishon Hawkins. In the course of research, I have visited several institutions and appreciate the librarians, archivists, and staff of the Moravian Archives of Salem, North Carolina; Newberry Library; Pennsylvania Historical Society; Haverford College Library; National Archives and Records Administration (Kansas City, Missouri, and Washington, D.C.); Library of Congress; Henry Huntington Library; American Philosophical Society; and William L. Clements Library. A number of libraries have provided digital images or photocopies of essential materials including the Thomas Gilcrease Museum; Pierpont Morgan Library; New York Public Library; David M. Rubenstein Rare Book & Manuscripts Library, Duke University; Museum of Early Southern Decorative Arts; and the Georgia Historical Society. I especially appreciate the following individuals for their kindly assistance: Olga Tsapina, Richard Starbuck, Brian Dunnigan, Renee Harvey, Ann Upton, Kate Collins, Lindsay Sheldon, Daniel Rolph, Lori Cox-Paul, Daisy Njoku, and Diana Sykes.

My research has been supported with financial support, release time, and opportunities to share my research provided by the University of Kansas. I began this project in earnest during a sabbatical leave in fall 2007. Special thanks go to the Hall Center for the Humanities for a Residential Fellowship, which provided me in spring 2008 with office space, a research grant, and a semester leave, while the College of Arts and Sciences awarded me General Research Fund grants (#2301136 and #2301031) and travel funds that kept this project going during my years as a department chair. Special thanks go to Ann Cudd, dean of Undergraduate Studies, whose crucial support at the end of the project expedited its completion. The Department of History provided travel and subvention funds as well as release time during 2013–14, without which the completion of this book would have been greatly delayed. It is my privilege to be in a department of accomplished scholars from whom I have learned a great deal. Special thanks go to Leslie Tuttle and Sheyda Jahanbani, who generously read and gave valuable feedback on various parts of the manuscript. I also appreciate the many colleagues and students who attended and offered their insights during presentations I made at the Peace, War, and Global Change Seminar at the Hall Center for the Humanities; the 23rd Annual James E. Seaver Lecture on Continuing Issues in Western Civilization, sponsored by the Humanities and Western Civilization Program; and the Annual Spring Lecture sponsored by the Indigenous Studies Program. I especially appreciate my fellow Cherokee specialist Michael Zogry for inviting me to give the latter talk and for the number of informal conversations about our shared intellectual interests.

Academic conferences and institutions other than my own have provided valuable opportunities to learn from others. I wish to thank my friends, colleagues, and students at nearby Haskell Indian Nations University, particularly Professor Eric Anderson, for allowing me to present my research to them. Aspects of this book were presented at the 2008 Indigenous Environments Seminar at Bowdoin College, Bowdoin, Maine; 2009 Mid-America History Conference, Norman, Oklahoma; and 2013 Beyond Germs Seminar at the Amerind Foundation, Dragoon, Arizona. My gratitude goes out to all of the participants in these programs and especially to David Gordon, Shepard Krech, Pekka Hämäläinen, Alan Swedlund, Catherine Cameron, David Jones, Robert Griswold, Laura Anderson, Gary Anderson, and Brad Raley. I have also engaged in a number of more informal discussions and e-mail chats with a number of generous individuals, some of whom supplied me microfilm, transcripts, and general information from their own ongoing research. Thank you, Robbie Ethridge, Greg Dowd, Phil Deloria, Peter Mancall, Joshua Piker, Steven Hahn, Brian Hosmer, Eric Hinderaker, and Wendy St. Jean. I have never met Alfred Crosby but this book would not be possible without his pioneering efforts, and although I offer alternatives to the "virgin soil" thesis, I respect his efforts to bring to light the ordeal that indigenous peoples faced after 1492, an ordeal that the general public seemed all too willing to forget at the time he began his career.

The production of this book has truly been a team effort. I worked with Darin Grauberger, Meghan Kelly, and KU's Cartographic Services to produce an excellent set of maps. The staff of the University of Oklahoma Press has been a joy to work with. Thank you Alessandra Tamulevich for sticking with this project and giving me encouragement at particularly needed times. The editorial assistance of a number of people has made this into a better book. The skilled copyediting of Susan Harris and thorough indexing of Mary Brooks brought this book to completion. Together this team kept me from making embarrassing mistakes, but those which remain are entirely due to my own oversight.

Given the subject matter, this work has been personally difficult at times. The Cherokee people both past and present have sustained me in my labors, and I owe them my sincere respect and gratitude. I had the good fortune of growing up in the small community of Chelsea, Oklahoma, a town within the current Cherokee Nation yet named after the much more famous area within London, England. I never fully understood this odd combination of Native and British worlds and probably never will, but researching this book has made me increasingly aware of the complicated colonial processes that have shaped the present realities of my family and community members. I wish I did not have to write this book, that a world existed for our indigenous ancestors in which colonial violence and germs did not exist, but since that world was a reality for several generations of Cherokees, I have endeavored to do my best to honor their legacy by setting the record straight and telling their story of survival.

To my family, I can never repay the love and support that I have received. My mother and father did not live to see the final result, but I know that they would be proud. My daughter Caroline has literally grown into a mature young woman as this project developed, and I am proud of her individual perseverance, especially during those times when I had to stay behind a computer to work. My wife, Stephanie, and I have shared a life together for ten years, a life full of shared hopes for a more just world and commitment to our wonderful children, Bradley and Katherine, who have filled me with more joy than I could have ever imagined. For making all of this possible, Stephanie, this book is dedicated to you.

CHEROKEE MEDICINE,
COLONIAL GERMS

INTRODUCTION

Smallpox, murder, and a cover-up. Mysterious circumstances set the stage for Savanukeh's visit to Coshocton at the height of the Revolutionary War. Savanukeh and fourteen of his fellow Cherokees arrived at the upper Ohio Valley town in June 1779 after traveling some three hundred miles from their Tennessee Valley homes. They had hoped to hear peace talks from Coshocton's pro-American Lenape headman, White Eyes. Instead, they found his people in a state of grief. White Eyes was dead. The Cherokees did as was expected of them and condoled with their mournful hosts. Savanukeh delivered a sorrowful yet healing talk, figuratively referencing White Eyes's absence and grave, "I observed yonder a dwelling closed up, and from which no smoke appeared to ascend. Looking in another direction, I discovered an elevated spot of fresh earth on which nothing was seen growing." Displaying his own sorrow, Savanukeh sat quietly for twenty minutes and then resumed his talk, now turning his efforts to assuaging the anguish of the Lenape. "See Grandfather," the Cherokee exclaimed using a kinship term to denote his hosts' status as the most ancient people of North America. "I level the ground on yonder spot of yellow earth and put leaves and brush thereon to make it invisible! I also sow seeds on that spot, so that both grass and trees may grow thereon." He handed the Lenape strings of beads and then reassured them: "Grandfather! The seed which I had sown has already taken root; nay, the grass has already covered the ground and the trees are growing!" He added at the end that "the cause of your grief being removed, let me dry up your tears!"[1] Throughout the three-hour ceremony, Savanukeh followed common Native protocol of not naming the deceased and his cause of death, a taboo that if violated would have ruinous consequences for a community's relations with the spirit world.

For different reasons, American officials remained mum as well, at least on paper. White Eyes had escorted Gen. Lachlan McIntosh and his troops on a fall 1778 mission to counter British influence among Native groups west of Coshocton, but as a consequence of this service White Eyes ended up in a grave back at Fort Pitt. McIntosh did not offer any written details of the Lenape leader's death and the only explanation from an American official that survives in the documentary record is that of Fort Pitt's commander, Col. Daniel Broadhead. In June 1779, Broadhead told the Lenape, "There was a great good Man called White Eyes. He was an honest man and a great counsellor but it was the will of God to call him to himself last fall."[2] Apparently, Broadhead and other officials verbally circulated a more specific account as well. "Capt. White Eyes . . . was taken with the smallpox, and was sent to Pittsburg where he soon died," a soldier later recalled while discussing the Ohio expedition.[3] The Christian missionary John Heckewelder, who worked at Coshocton and recorded Savanukeh's condolence talk, recorded the same story in his memoirs. White Eyes, according to Heckewelder, wanted "a general peace" but "did not live to see that day, for while accompanying general M'Intosh's army . . . he took the smallpox and died."[4] The American agent George Morgan knew otherwise. Morgan, who was stationed at Fort Pitt during the revolution, later wrote to Congress in 1784 that White Eyes "was treacherously put to death at the moment of his greatest exertions to serve the United States."[5] American militiamen, Morgan's testimony appears to suggest and most historians concur, executed the Lenape leader and high-ranking officials covered up the death.

Americans at the time certainly had no reason to doubt that White Eyes had died of smallpox. The virus seemed to be everywhere during the American Revolution and had a history of doing particular harm to indigenous peoples.[6] White Eyes's Euro-American contemporaries were surely aware of what many readers of this book probably already know: European colonization unleashed tragic epidemiological consequences for indigenous peoples. Smallpox especially found its way into Native communities, caused appalling casualties, and figured prominently in the records colonizers produced for the literate world. The Spanish, for example, produced vivid accounts of what the disease did after its first documented introduction to the Americas in 1518 and its subsequent spread to Mexico in 1520. One participant in Cortez's conquest of the Aztecs recorded, "When the Christians were exhausted from war God saw fit to send the Indians smallpox, and there was a great pestilence. . . . We soldiers could scarcely get about the streets because of the Indians who were sick from hunger, pestilence and smallpox."[7] The English also referenced a terrible outbreak during the formative stage of the Massachusetts Bay Colony. In 1634, Gov. John Winthrop reported, "But for the natives in these parts, God hath so pursued them, as for 300 miles space the greatest part of them are swept away by the smallpox which still continues among them. So as God hath thereby cleared our title to this place."[8] Another round of the disease swept the American South in the 1690s as the English struggled to establish its colonies of North and South Carolina. Governor John Archdale said of his indigenous neighbors: "The Hand of God was eminently seen in thinning the Indians to make room for the English. . . . But again, it at other times pleased Almighty God to send unusual sicknesses amongst them, as the smallpox, &c. to lessen their numbers."[9] Just as Archdale had echoed colonists before him, his successors would perpetuate his conclusions—conclusions that had become widely familiar to White Eyes's American contemporaries: indigenous peoples had a traumatic experience with smallpox that occurred outside of the control of Europeans and that aided the newcomers in their quest to acquire land and build colonies.[10]

Scholars today generally agree with these conclusions as well. Instead of their colonial predecessors' theological explanations, however, they have largely adopted the "virgin soil" thesis that historian Alfred Crosby has most cogently developed. Indigenous peoples, Crosby maintains, fell victim to not just smallpox but a litany of diseases that they had no prior experience with and were "therefore immunologically almost defenseless." The defenses—the antibodies that are created after surviving an infectious disease—were absent not because of any genetic weakness that Natives possessed and certainly not because of any divine favoritism for Europeans. Instead, several deadly diseases were simply not in the Americas until their introductions after 1492. Thereafter, waves of novel germs found their way into Native communities in which everyone lacked antibodies and in which nearly universal infection or "virgin soil" epidemics occurred. As Crosby states, "The initial appearance of these diseases is as certain to have set off deadly epidemics as dropping lighted matches into tinder is certain to cause fires." The germs even outpaced the colonizers. Crosby maintains that diseases spread beyond the purview of literate observers, igniting outbreaks that went unrecorded, as "many of the most important events of aboriginal history in British America occurred beyond the range of direct observation by literate witnesses."[11]

Crosby's "virgin soil" thesis not only explains why diseases spread so fast over great distances but also proposes why extreme mortality occurred during epidemics. One must first realize that the germs introduced, particularly the smallpox virus, caused a serious and potentially lethal illness that could not be cured. During the colonial era, smallpox ordinarily killed a proportion of the people it infected, among all racial and ethnic groups. When it struck previously unexposed populations, however, it afflicted all age groups—not just children or those relatively few adults that managed to escape infection during childhood as happened in Europe. A collapse of social services within an initially stricken community subsequently occurred and mortality rates soared. Men and women in the prime of their life became desperately ill, leaving no one to care for the sick, acquire food, and protect from enemies. Indigenous populations also faced waves of epidemics. Colonization introduced multiple diseases that in some instances struck Native communities simultaneously and in other instances in rapid succession. Subsequent episodes of the same disease, moreover, occurred because the most virulent germs such as smallpox quickly ran out of susceptible victims, disappeared for up to a decade or more, and then after being reintroduced by colonizers returned to indigenous communities to strike those born after the previous epidemic. Finally, Native responses to epidemics drove up mortality. Crosby argues that "traditional customs and religions though perhaps effective against pre-Columbian diseases, were rarely so against acute infections from abroad, and they were often dangerous as in the swift transfer of a patient from broiling sweathouse to frigid lake." Natives also supposedly "had no conception of contagion and did not practice quarantine of the sick in pre-Columbian times, nor did they accept the new theory or practice until taught to do so by successive disasters." This "ignorance" led to frenzied, destructive behavior such as suicides, abandonment of the sick, and flight to other communities, thereby spreading contagion even more thoroughly. These responses, Crosby concludes, proved as significant in causing mortality as did the virulence of the germ itself.[12]

The "virgin soil" thesis thus places great weight on a historical accident—European colonization's unintended introduction of diseases to a previously unexposed indigenous population—and to the inability of Natives to deal effectively with the epidemiological crises that ensued. The colonizers exercised little agency in this catastrophe yet were its unwitting beneficiaries. Crosby and others, to be sure, do not deny that "warfare, murder, [and] dispossession" occurred and that these contributed to depopulation. Nevertheless, smallpox and its deadly companions were enough to facilitate conquest. Or as Crosby stated in his highly acclaimed book, *Ecological Imperialism:* "It was their germs, not these imperialists themselves, for all of their brutality and callousness, that were chiefly responsible for sweeping aside indigenes and opening the [Americas] to demographic takeover."[13]

Such a conclusion has reverberated throughout the pages of both academic and popular works of history. The anthropologist Henry Dobyns, in particular, published works on Native American demography that both influenced and were influenced by the "virgin soil" thesis. Dobyns maintained that early Euro-Americans "had good reason to suppose that Native Americans would disappear" because of the "simple reason" that "Old World pathogens . . . escaped from their original hosts to invade new territory." Beginning no later than 1520, a series of pandemics swept the Western Hemisphere, leaving North America a "widowed" continent by the time of Euro-American settlement.[14] Dobyns's postulation of these undocumented pandemics supports a goal he set as early as 1966 to convince his colleagues that the Americas' aboriginal population in 1492 could have been as high as 112 million, a much larger number than an upper limit of 14 million that many anthropologist seemed willing to accept at the time.[15] Jared Diamond supported such a high count and relied heavily on Crosby's and Dobyns's scholarship in his Pulitzer Prize–winning interpretation of global history, *Guns, Germs, and Steel: The Fates of Human Societies*. He writes, "As for the most advanced native societies of North America . . . their destruction was accomplished largely by germs alone, introduced by early European explorers and advancing ahead of them."[16] Similarly, Charles Mann in *1491: New Revelations of the Americas before Columbus*, which won the National Academy of Science's Keck Award for best book of the year award, claimed that Native "societies were destroyed by weapons their opponents could not control and did not even know they had."[17] Europeans were the opponents, and diseases served as their unwitting weapons. "Colonial writers knew that disease tilled the virgin soil of the Americas countless times in the sixteenth century," he writes. "But what they did not, could not, know is that the epidemics shot out like ghastly arrows from the limited areas they saw to every corner of the hemisphere, wreaking destruction in places that never appeared in the European historical record."[18]

The lived realities of individuals such as Savanukeh, however, suggest different conclusions. Not only did smallpox serve as a cover-up in the death of the Lenape leader he traveled so far to see, but from a larger perspective the disease has played a role in historical interpretations that obscures more than illuminates. Savanukeh remained silent on what he thought caused White Eyes's death—we cannot know whether he believed the stories that Americans circulated—but we do know what he had to say about the circumstances of his own people. When he journeyed home from Coshocton, the Cherokees were rebuilding their nation shattered by prior American invasions, facing exposure to smallpox as it followed the course of the Revolutionary War into the South, and grappling with difficult choices: Do they remain allied to King George III, whose armies possibly could drive the Americans into submission, or do they reject their British alliance, cease reprisals against settlers, and hope that passivity will save them from further destruction? Cherokees made different choices; some sought vengeance against the settlers, while others sought to appease the Americans. All suffered the consequences for being seen as British allies. According to Savanukeh, reporting about a series of American invasions in 1780 and 1781, "The Rebels from Virginia attacked . . . in such numbers there was no withstanding them, they dyed their hands in the Blood of our Women and Children, burnt 17 towns, destroyed all our provisions by which we & our families were almost destroyed by famine this spring."[19] While detailing the murder of his people, he made no mention of smallpox, although historians have claimed the disease to have inflicted a deadly blow on the Cherokees in 1780.[20]

Savanukeh's words point to a much darker and troubling view of the past, one in which the independent actions of germs do not serve as the chief determinant in the transition of the Americas from indigenous to European control. Epidemics, to be sure, occurred, but as this book intends to show, scholars have overlooked how colonialism's violence set the stage for these supposedly unintended biological events, curtailed the abilities of Natives to protect themselves from infection, exacerbated mortality, and impeded recovery. Modern historians of course are not deliberately engaged in a conscious effort to deny that violent deaths of untold numbers of indigenous peoples occurred; the "virgin soil" thesis was not crafted as an apology for the colonizers, and it still has some utility in explaining how history has unfolded. It has, however, unfortunately hidden colonialism's violence under a cloak of biological determinism.

• • • •

This book thus aims to remove this cloak and focus on how human agency shaped the experience of indigenous peoples with colonialism's most deadly germ, smallpox. Focusing on just one Native group—the Cherokee Nation—might appear to limit this book's challenge to the conclusions of the "virgin soil" thesis. Nevertheless, an exclusive focus is exactly what is called for in the study of introduced diseases and their impact on indigenous peoples. Studies that have had the most influence on both scholarly and popular interpretations paint with large brush strokes, take a broad look at regions or continents, and make sweeping generalizations based on unconnected anecdotes. Historians too often take written accounts such as those of Winthrop and Archdale out of their immediate context and uncritically accept each as illustrating a universal phenomenon. Modern scholars, moreover, have generally overlooked how such accounts built on each other. Both Winthrop and Archdale, for example, almost certainly had read about the Spanish conquest of the Aztecs and came to their respective colonies already prepared to interpret what epidemiological consequences would occur. The documentary record then becomes filled with smallpox epidemics that happened for a limited set of reasons and that involved powerless Native victims and innocent European bystanders. In the end, colonial accounts created a powerful narrative that gave germs agency in the destruction of Native peoples, blamed the victims for their incompetent response to those germs, and thereby exonerated colonizers from responsibility. An in-depth study of one indigenous group's experience with smallpox, though, can reveal a much more complicated story, one in which each supposed account is put into a larger historical context and subjected to critical analysis to determine whether it represented what actually happened or only what the writer imagined to have happened.[21]

The Cherokees serve as a most appropriate subject for such a study. Their nation already figures prominently in the scholarly literature due to a particularly vivid and widely cited passage from James Adair's *The History of the American Indians* (originally published in London in 1775). Adair, a British trader who worked among the southeastern Natives from the 1730s into the 1760s, detailed the Cherokees' first documented encounter with smallpox: "About the year 1738, the Cherokee received a most depopulating shock by the smallpox, which reduced them almost one half, in about a year's time."[22] He further describes a chaotic and horrid scene that modern scholars have seized upon to illustrate how Native healers responded ineffectually to epidemics, concluding that the Cherokee medical personnel proved "deficient in proper skill" to halt what to them was a "foreign" and "strange" disease and took measures that proved deadly to their patients and to themselves. Healers, the trader claimed, had their patients heat themselves to a sweat and then plunge into the nearby river, a practice that led to immediate death. The bewildered doctors "broke their old consecrated physic pots, and threw away all other pretended holy things they had for physical use, imagining they had lost their divine power by being polluted." He adds that a "great many" physicians chose to share the fate of their patients and committed suicide. "Some shot themselves, others cut their throats, some stabbed themselves with knives, and others with sharp-pointed canes; many threw themselves with sullen madness into the fire, and there slowly expired, as if they had been utterly divested of the native power of feeling pain."[23] It would seem, then, that Adair's account provides a unique window through which to view how indigenous peoples responded to smallpox.

James Adair's account can tell us much—and it will be subjected to much more analysis later in this book—but the point of choosing the Cherokee Nation as a case study is not because of this one single passage. Instead, with this nation, a scholar has much more to base his or her findings on than anecdotal evidence. From their location at the southern end of the Appalachian Mountains, the Cherokees emerged in the early eighteenth century as one the most prominent indigenous polities to exercise power during the colonial era. While consisting of dozens of largely autonomous villages arrayed in four geographical clusters, Cherokees possessed a degree of unity through mutually intelligible dialects of an Iroquoian language, kinship connections through a system of seven matrilineal clans, military cooperation against common enemies, and a shared alliance with Great Britain. The indigenous nation supplied the colonies of Virginia and South Carolina with deerskins and slaves in exchange for guns, ammunition, cloth, and other manufactured items and frequently offered the British military assistance against Native, French, and then their American enemies. After the revolution, Cherokees came to serve as a focal point in the development of U.S. Indian policy. They appeared to accept American demands to conform to Euro-American culture by coalescing into a more centralized republic, transitioning to commercial agriculture, and welcoming Christian missionaries to open schools and churches in their midst. This intensive relationship with the British and then the Americans unfortunately led to documented outbreaks of smallpox among them but also a particularly rich documentary record to reconstruct those experiences. Correspondence, reports, and memoirs of numerous traders, missionaries, government officials, and visitors reveal the complicated context in which disease spread, illustrate varied and evolving responses to epidemics, and highlight how the violence of colonialism affected Native efforts to recover from successive bouts of smallpox. Such relatively voluminous evidence indicates that Cherokee leaders incorporated smallpox into their cosmology, constructed rituals to deal with threatened or actual epidemics of the disease, and gave constructive advice to their followers about avoiding exposure. Adair's passage in other words is not all there is to understand how Cherokees experienced smallpox.[24] A richer and more varied array of sources demonstrate that Cherokees put up a sustained fight against colonialism's most dangerous germ, a germ that current historiography renders as too powerful for Natives even to try to combat.

An exclusive examination of Cherokee history then mobilizes multiple and varied sources that bring into question interpretations based on anecdotal-type evidence. Similarly, there are important reasons for putting the smallpox virus or *Variola major* at the center of this book's analysis. At the time of colonization, *Variola* caused one of the deadliest illnesses known to humanity. Victims stood a 40 percent chance of dying from the disease or an even greater chance if their health had been compromised by malnourishment or simultaneous occurrence of multiple diseases. People contracted this deadly germ through inhalation but would not know they had the disease for ten to fourteen days during which time the virus incubated. After this period ended, excruciating symptoms occurred. Victims first suffered extremely high fevers, ones that could reach deadly levels and kill people before they knew what disease they had. About the fourth day, the characteristic pustules erupted. These painful sores began on the face and then spread over the trunk and appendages. The eyes were particularly vulnerable to pustules, as these could form around the eye socket and cause permanent blindness. Pustules also could rupture underneath the skin and cause an individual to bleed to death. For about ten days a smallpox victim's body was a grotesque site, a swollen mess with numerous pus-filled and bloody lesions. For those fortunate to survive, recovery started around the fourteenth

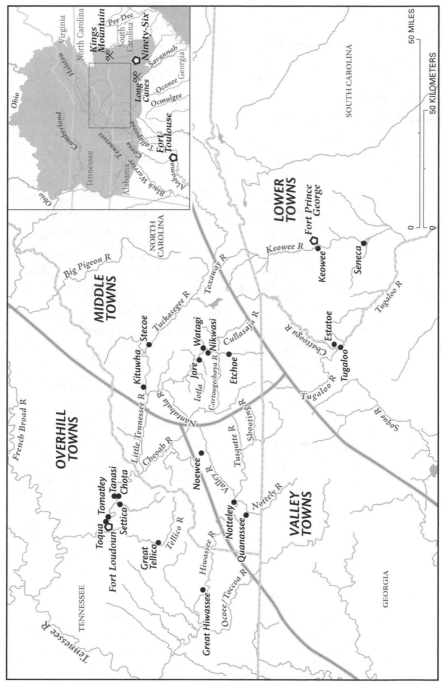

Cherokee Nation prior to American Revolution. Map by Darin Grauberger and Meghan Kelly, University of Kansas Cartographic Services.

day after the fever began. Then, no new pustules emerged and the old ones began to heal. These would scab over and eventually fall off, often leaving the skin forever scarred or pitted.[25]

Smallpox, to be sure, was not the only highly lethal disease that accompanied Europeans and Africans to the Americas. Other acute infectious diseases—or those that induce a rapid onset of symptoms and do not persist in the body for extended periods—arrived on American shores repeatedly after 1492 and proved deadly to indigenous peoples. But among this list of killers, smallpox stood out. That European observers could most easily recognize smallpox's gruesome characteristics explains in part why that disease received the most attention; colonists lived in an early modern world in which those who were untrained in what at the time was rather limited medical knowledge often referred to other diseases in general terms such as "pestilential fevers" and "distempers." Still, there were other, more important, reasons that made smallpox most significant. Compared to other acute infectious diseases of a lethal nature, smallpox had a comparatively lengthy period of incubation and communicability and thus could travel greater distances. A victim could harbor the incubating virus for ten to fourteen days and then shed it through exhalation for about a two-week period. The virus also could remain viable up to two more weeks within the scabs it formed, making a nonimmune person vulnerable to contracting the disease through close contact with those scabs. Scabs could adhere to blankets, bedding, bandages, and clothing thus putting any nonimmune person who handled such objects in jeopardy. It is also possible that the virus survived by itself for up to a year on woolen or cloth material in cool and dry conditions; such limitations, however, made its spread by such means problematic and lead us to believe that the disease spread in most cases through direct human-to-human contact or through materials contaminated with recent scabs. Still, the virus remained viable for a much longer period than a whole host of other diseases thought to have accompanied Europeans or Africans to the Americas.[26] Influenza, for example, incubates for one to two days and thereafter is communicable for three to five days.[27] Measles has a period of incubation and direct communicability equivalent to that of smallpox, but it must be passed directly from person-to-person by way of exhalation and inhalation.[28] Certainly, influenza and measles epidemics struck indigenous peoples. Smallpox, though, more often spread beyond the point of initial contact between Natives and newcomers and erupted into outbreaks much more massive in scale.

The practice of variolation also helps explain why smallpox became the most significant disease to plague indigenous peoples. This procedure involved the deliberate inoculation of someone with smallpox matter harvested from the pustules or scabs of another person suffering from an active case of the disease. The purpose of variolation was to produce in the inoculated person a more mild and survivable form of the disease. The practice had been known in Asia and Africa for some time and caught on in Great Britain and her American colonies in the second and third decades of the eighteenth century. A variolater usually transmitted the infection through an incision on the patient's hand or arm. If all went well, the patient began to display relatively weak symptoms—low-grade fever and minor pustules that could serve as a source of smallpox matter for others to be inoculated with. Sometimes the procedure did not go as planned, however, and the more virulent form of the disease and even death resulted. Variolaters, moreover, did not always practice strict quarantine of their patients. Even those who had the mild form of the disease were contagious and could transfer *Variola* to a nonimmune person through natural means, thus giving that person the deadlier form of the disease.

Variolation thus remained controversial throughout the eighteenth century as it caused deaths and fueled smallpox outbreaks. Its unregulated practice made epidemics more widespread than they ordinarily would have been and thus increased the opportunities for a dreaded germ to reach distant and remote indigenous villages. The practice ultimately was discarded with the discovery of, and should not be confused with, the newer and much safer procedure of vaccination. Most famously promoted by the English physician Edward Jenner in 1798, vaccination involved the deliberate inoculation of an individual with cowpox—a virus that produces only minor skin eruptions yet induces the body's immune system to produce antibodies that shield one from the genetically similar smallpox. This revolutionary procedure put humanity on course to ultimately eradicate a disease that had brought so much death and suffering, and its introduction to the Cherokees serves as the focus of this book's last chapter. Until then, though, Western medical procedures offered little to curtail the spread of smallpox, and variolation actually escalated its circulation among North American populations.

Variola also spread more easily and widely than many other acute germs because of a relative lack of environmental prerequisites for its transmission. Smallpox did not depend on an insect vector or intermediary animal host. Some extremely deadly diseases thought to have been shipped to the Americas do have such prerequisites. Humans can contract the yellow fever virus, for example, when bitten by an infected mosquito belonging to the species *Aedes aegypti*. These mosquitoes, though, remain restricted to waterfront areas and live permanently only in locations where the temperature remains above seventy-one degrees Fahrenheit. Major yellow fever epidemics did occur in colonial North America but these involved the introduction of both the virus and mosquito to urban port cities during the warm season.[29] Since such outbreaks could not and did not spread far inland, the Cherokees were only vulnerable to yellow fever if they traveled to the seacoast at an inopportune time. Bubonic plague's arrival in North America was even more problematic and perhaps not possible until the development of steam ships in the nineteenth century. Certain species of fleas transmit the plague bacteria to a human host. The bacteria then incubate two to six days and remain contagious for no more than a week. Plague, of course, is extremely lethal—even more so than smallpox—but since it often killed its victim within a matter of days, its spread remained much more limited. Historic epidemics of plague in fact have depended in large measure on rodent populations that can harbor the disease. In the case of the famous Black Death in fourteenth-century Europe, plague became transmitted to black rats that commonly infested the dwellings of an increasingly urban Europe. It is doubtful that wind-powered ships made the Atlantic passage quickly enough for plague to persist within either a human or rat population, and even if plague did arrive on the shores of North America sometime during the colonial era, the bacteria likely did not find a population living in dense enough concentrations and with the necessary flea and rodent vectors to ignite a massive outbreak.[30] Similarly, typhus—a serious but not as deadly disease as plague—depended on lice and fleas. Typhus epidemics have historically been associated with peoples forced to live in unsanitary conditions such as urban slums or large army encampments. Transatlantic ships certainly had such conditions, and typhus likely did make several passages to North America, but once it arrived, it did not spread to Natives as easily as did smallpox, given the relatively dispersed and clean living conditions of indigenous peoples.[31]

Some diseases, to be sure, did spread as thoroughly as did smallpox, but these were considerably less deadly. Typhoid fever, for example, became a fairly widespread disease during the colonial period. The bacteria that cause this disease may have existed in the Americas before 1492 but a pre-Columbian presence remains uncertain.[32] What is certain is that colonial settlement facilitated outbreaks of the disease. Infected victims pass the disease onto others when their urine and fecal matter contaminates the water or food supply of others. Typhoid victims can shed the bacteria for varying lengths of time. Most will do so for about a month, but 10 percent of victims can carry the disease up to three months while 2 to 5 percent can become permanent carriers. Such longevity made the disease easy to transmit across the Atlantic and across the continent. The disease caused quite unpleasant symptoms—headaches, sustained fevers, despondency, anorexia, slowness of heartbeat, enlargement of the spleen, cough, rose-colored spots on the body, and bowel problems—but an individual's likelihood of dying paled in comparison to smallpox. Typhoid has a case fatality rate of 10 percent among untreated victims.[33]

Chronic infectious diseases also spread widely but could not have produced the catastrophic mortality that smallpox did. Maladies in this category persist in the body much longer than the acute variety. In general, they have been ancient infections of humanity and have consequently evolved into mild infections. It is in the germ's interest in fact not to kill its human host too quickly; the germ must be passed on to others in order to continue replicating and thus perpetuate itself as a species. Some of these highly evolved diseases such as tuberculosis, syphilis, and hepatitis B likely infected our hunter-gatherer ancestors and persisted in most populations across the globe, including American Natives, before 1492. Cherokees indeed were not disease free prior to the arrival of Europeans. Their bodies served as hosts not only to the highly evolved pathogens listed above but also to a variety of chronic infections involving fungi, bacteria, and worms that all humans have had to endure.[34]

One chronic infectious disease, however, that was certainly imported to the Americas after 1492 was malaria. Caused by protozoa belonging to the species *Plasmodium*, malaria depends on *Anopheles* mosquitoes for its transmission to humans. After an infected mosquito injects it into a human host, *Plasmodia* invade the human body and can reside there for a year or even longer, causing periodic cycles of chills and fevers, headaches, nausea, and profuse sweating. Since the disease persists so long in the human body, the disease readily journeyed across the Atlantic and became seeded in the Americas wherever human carriers traveled into areas infested with *Anopheles*. These pests indeed lived in the Americas before 1492 and could be found in their preferred habitat—areas with slow-moving or stagnant waterways with a nearby mammal population upon which to feed. Permanent Native settlements near swamps, oxbow lakes, or meandering rivers proved especially vulnerable to malaria. Still, malaria's symptoms generally debilitate but do not kill people. The most typical form of malaria has a case fatality rate of less than 10 percent for untreated victims, making it significantly less traumatic for indigenous peoples than smallpox.[35]

As traumatic as smallpox was, however, one need not assume that indigenous peoples were genetically predisposed to die from the disease. Unfortunately, many scholars have misinterpreted Crosby's "virgin soil" thesis to imply Native genetic inferiority, despite his warnings against such conclusion.[36] Human bodies across the globe responded to smallpox in the same way. For first-time victims, white blood cells detected the presence of the foreign virus and produced antibodies specifically designed to render the germ harmless, and for all first-time victims, such a response was ineffective. The production of antibodies could not keep up with the replication of the virus, which essentially hijacked the body and induced symptoms that then facilitated its spread to a new victim. Fortunately, antibodies to smallpox stayed in the body after the disease ran its course and were immediately available to attack and destroy the virus when reintroduced. Sometimes infants were born with a degree of acquired immunity due to antibodies they received from their mother while in the womb or from their mothers' breast milk. Such immunity did not last, and children eventually became susceptible to smallpox. Of course, in 1492 no indigenous person possessed antibodies to fight smallpox, making for a potentially explosive situation when the virus eventually reached unexposed communities. Consequent epidemics, though, were the result of a general lack of acquired immunity and not a result of bad genes.

Genetic immunity to infectious diseases rarely exists. It refers to specific inherited traits that give an individual a better chance to avoid a disease or suffer less than an individual who lacks those inherited traits. Such an advantage only develops after tens of thousands of years of natural selection and involves only a relatively few diseases that are among the oldest known to humans. The sickle cell trait, for example, is an advantage against malaria, giving individuals who carry these genes the ability to fight off malaria. This advantage has led to high rates of sickle cell carriers among populations that have had a long exposure to malaria. The increased number of these carriers of course comes with its own problems. Individuals who inherit the genes from both of their parents develop the irregularly shaped red blood cells that inhibit blood flow, cause anemia, and result in a number of other problems, including stroke at an early age. Unlike malaria, smallpox has not been a human infection long enough for natural selection to produce any known genetic advantages. The disease emerged from a mutated virus endemic within cattle populations around six thousand years ago after human beings began keeping domestic livestock. Smallpox thus has afflicted no more than two hundred generations, a small blip in the entire trajectory of human evolution. During the era of colonization, European children were dying at alarming rates. One study even claims that

80 percent of London's children younger than five years of age who became infected with smallpox during the eighteenth century did not survive the disease.[37]

Rather than genetics and even the universal absence of acquired immunity to smallpox that characterized indigenous societies before 1518, human agency played a determinative and unmistakable role in shaping the contours of death and survival of indigenous peoples during their long struggle with colonialism. Each of the five following chapters, while organized chronologically, focuses on uncovering the choices and actions of people that underlay the Cherokees' experiences with smallpox. The story begins with a long false dawn between 1518 and the mid-sixteenth century when sporadic encounters with Europeans did little to bring Cherokees into the wider circulation of guns, goods, and germs that were beginning to transform Native worlds. By the 1690s the story becomes more intense as English-inspired slave raids triggered a massive smallpox epidemic that likely struck the Cherokees for the first time. As the eighteenth century wore on, Cherokees continually had to respond to real and threatened epidemics and did so with some effectiveness by drawing on their own medicine. Yet they also faced terribly destructive physical violence with the British Empire during the Anglo-Cherokee War (1759–61) and American militias during the Revolutionary War (1775–83). After suffering much more from the scourge of warfare than smallpox, Cherokees rebounded during the early nineteenth century and took part in the nascent global effort to eradicate *Variola* by embracing vaccine in 1824. In doing so, Cherokees by no means dispensed with their Native medical practices and beliefs. This story of *Variola* and its Native victims is thus a more complicated story than their supposedly ill-equipped bodies and counterproductive responses. The lived experiences of Savanukeh and his fellow Cherokees exemplify this complexity and demonstrate how Europeans and their American descendants have obscured the past with the accounts they left behind and how contemporary historians perpetuate a simplistic understanding of conquest with the "virgin soil" thesis.

CHAPTER 1

ARRIVAL

Smallpox raced ahead of colonizers, reached many Natives before they had even seen Europeans, and caused catastrophic yet undocumented epidemics, or at least that it is what the figurative language that pervades the historical literature attempts to demonstrate. "The disease spread like wildfire through a Native American population that was 100 percent susceptible," Dobyns asserts about smallpox.[1] Crosby similarly compares colonial germs to "matches" and Native bodies to "tinder," to call up an image of disease conflagrations, engulfing indigenous peoples with inextinguishable fury.[2] Later, he uses a metaphor drawn from European folklore to champion Dobyns's idea of an early hemispheric pandemic of *Variola*. "Smallpox is a disease with seven-league boots," he writes in reference to magical footwear that allows wearers to cover great distances speedily with each stride taken.[3] Mann uses a colorful simile, when postulating that smallpox "radiated" through the Incan Empire "like ink spreading through tissue paper" before Pizarro began his conquest.[4] James Axtell, a prolific historian of Native North America, employs a more militaristic metaphor when suggesting that indigenous peoples suffered in advance of actual colonization. Axtell characterizes smallpox as "microbic shock troops which swept unseen through defenseless Indian villages with lethal ruthlessness, reducing dramatically the natives' numerical superiority."[5] David Kennedy and his coauthors in their popular college textbook choose a completely different depiction. "Lethal germs spread among the New World peoples with the speed and force of a hurricane," the *American Pageant* teaches its students, "swiftly sweeping far ahead of the human invaders."[6] Such vivid imagery has much interpretive appeal: it lures readers to believe that nothing existed to stop smallpox once Europeans inadvertently introduced it to an inexperienced Native population.

Such characterizations also lead one to assume that the virus must have initially arrived among Cherokees before its first documented occurrence in 1738. But when? The Cherokees had been engaged in sustained trading with the English since the late 1690s and small-pox broke out in the nearby colonies of Virginia and South Carolina in 1696, 1711, and 1718. Colonial officials and settlers took note of its impact on a variety of Native groups, except Cherokees who would remain unmentioned as victims but who nonetheless may have been infected.[7] Colonialism's most dreaded disease may have reached them even earlier. To the north, *Variola* arrived in the 1630s, spreading westward from the recently established Massachusetts Bay Colony to the Five Nations or Iroquois Confederacy in what is today upstate New York and then traveling even farther to encompass the peoples of the Great Lakes.[8] Around the same time, colonial germs devas-tated thousands of Natives of Spanish Florida. Introduced diseases spread within a Catholic mission system that by 1630 stretched north-ward from Saint Augustine to near the Savannah River and westward to the Apalachicola River.[9] Another possibility even more distant in time is that sixteenth-century Spanish explorers directly introduced smallpox to Cherokees. Two separate Spanish expeditions, one led by Hernando de Soto in 1540 and the other by Juan Pardo in 1567, crossed the mountains near where Cherokees were located in the eighteenth century. But perhaps *Variola* beat them there. In 1518 and 1519, smallpox struck Spain's Caribbean Island colonies and then traveled to Mexico where it sparked a massive outbreak among the Aztecs. During the early 1520s, it possibly spread through a univer-sally vulnerable population from Canada to Chile.[10] As one goes back further in time, more opportunities seem to exist for smallpox to have caused one or more epidemics among Cherokees that Europeans did not record.

It must be remembered, however, that no matter how many scena-rios existed for smallpox to make an undocumented arrival, each one remained only a *possibility*. Conclusive evidence cannot be marshaled to prove that smallpox arrived for the first time among Cherokees as late as 1718 or as early as the 1520s or sometime in between. But, what can be developed is a *most likely* scenario. To do this, one must eschew the metaphors and other literary devices that figure so prominently in the "virgin soil" literature. These oversimplify how and why epidemics actually occurred. Colonialism's most dangerous germ did not have wings that magically propelled it from place to place but instead depended on a chain of human-to-human contacts; with any break in this chain, the virus found no more hosts, its replication stopped, and the epidemic burned out. In order for an indigenous group to have an encounter with the deadly disease, their communities had to be a link in a continuous communication network that stretched from the place of smallpox's introduction. Settlement patterns, political organization, trading practices, warfare, and other characteristics of aboriginal society that affected a particular group's connections with the outside world must be considered. The issues in determining smallpox's arrival to a particular group thus become far more complicated.

A lack of acquired immunity alone in other words cannot account for indigenous susceptibility. The "virgin soil" concept obscures vast differences among indigenous societies that scholars must take into account. Some Natives lived in empires with hundreds of thousands of people; others lived in small independent towns with only hundreds. Some had extensive trading ties that brought foreign items into their communities from great distances; others had little involvement with exchange outside of their immediate location. Some groups moved hundreds of miles in search of food; others lived in permanent settlements and made only short trips from their residences. The notion of "virginity" also homogenizes the varied experiences Natives had with colonialism. Some had their lives quickly and dramatically changed through military conquest, enslavement, trade, or missionary activity; others felt colonialism's effects more gradually and piecemeal. All of these factors—both aboriginal and colonial—played roles in determining the timing and impact of smallpox's arrival.

While investigating these multiple issues can only lead to most likely yet still nondefinitive answers, there is much importance in addressing them. The interpretive stakes are high. On one hand, if an indigenous group suffered an epidemic soon after 1518 and experienced repeated bouts with *Variola* before its members developed regular and sustained relations with nearby Europeans, then germs and not the colonizers themselves were overwhelmingly responsible for the depopulation that occurred. In the case of the Cherokees, this would mean that the 10,379 Cherokees that the British counted in 1721 represented only a shattered shell of their Nation as it existed before European contact.[11] On the other hand, if smallpox did not arrive until after Europeans established a presence near a particular indigenous group and consequently altered its members' way of life, then germs played a less independent role, one necessarily tied to the broader aspects of colonialism including trading, warfare, and diplomacy. In this case, the overall depopulation would have been of a smaller magnitude but the agency of the colonizers would deserve more scrutiny.

• • • •

Metaphoric and hyperbolic characterizations of smallpox's first introduction obscures vast differences among Native societies, differences that must be taken into account when considering any possible chain of infection that facilitated a hemispheric smallpox pandemic in the 1520s. Then, *Variola* found in central Mexico the densely populated Aztecan Empire and consequently sparked a massive epidemic. The capital of Tenochtitlan alone held some two hundred thousand to three hundred thousand people in which a contagious disease could easily spread. The virus also found its way outside of the city into the Aztec's subordinate dominions. A system of tribute and military rule kept these subordinates closely connected to their leaders and thus provided the necessary traffic to transmit smallpox from the center to the peripheries of the empire.[12] Documentary evidence, although with some ambiguity regarding the symptoms and exact timing, also indicates that the pandemic devastated the Mayans of Central America and reached the Isthmus of Panama. Given the Mayans' location, their extensive trading activities, and their homeland being among the most densely populated areas in the Americas, they certainly were vulnerable to contracting the epidemic and sustaining a major epidemic.[13] Some evidence points to smallpox's spread even farther to the south. Although with some dissent, scholars generally believe that the pandemic reached the Incas, a populous and expansive empire that dominated the Andean Mountain chain from Ecuador to Chile.[14] Scholars give less support to *Variola*'s spread northward out of central Mexico. The virus certainly made it as far as the Tarascan Empire of Michoacán, but beyond there its spread would have become increasingly improbable. Geographic barriers such as deserts, swamps, and mountains posed discontinuities in human communication, while populations became sparser and trading ties became weaker.[15]

Even if smallpox made it to the Rio Grande or to the shores of the Gulf or Atlantic Coast in the 1520s, the likelihood that the pandemic continued to spread through the remainder of the North American continent appears negligible. No polities such as the Tarascan, Aztecan, or Incan empires existed within what becomes the United States. Most people living in the Southeast, for example, belonged to simple chiefdoms. These polities generally consisted of four or five towns united together under the leadership of a central community and an elite that may have inherited its status. This central community usually had at least one earthen mound where priests oversaw activities such as fertility, military, and mortuary rituals that held the chiefdom together. Priests did not rule with military force as did leaders in states but instead used religious persuasion. They were believed to have sacred knowledge that allowed their followers to have abundant harvests, military successes, and good health.[16] Typical chiefdoms occupied about twenty kilometers of territory and had villages with populations ranging between 350 and 650 people, making a total polity population of 2,800 to 5,400.[17] Sometimes simple chiefdoms allied with others for mutual defense and cooperation, and sometimes these alliances developed into paramount chiefdoms. One of these polities once existed at Cahokia, just east of present-day Saint Louis. At its height in the twelfth century, Cahokia contained 120 mounds arrayed over 1,600 hectares. Multiple communities and tens of thousands of people living in the highly fertile area of southern Illinois paid homage to Cahokia's leaders. Cahokia, however, was exceptional in scale and complexity. It also collapsed before 1492. At the time smallpox ravaged the Aztecs, no other polity in the Eastern Woodlands came close to possessing Cahokia's size and complexity.[18]

The Cherokees, in particular, had little vulnerability to an infectious disease introduced at a faraway location. They remained a collection of independent simple chiefdoms with limited connections to the world outside of their rugged mountainous homeland. Their towns were economically redundant and self-sufficient. That is each community relied on the same set of activities to produce food, and each produced enough to feed its own residents. Women cultivated fields of maize, beans, and squash that provided the majority of calories that their respective communities consumed, while men brought in the bulk of protein through hunting. White-tailed deer supplied the most meat, while turkeys, bears, squirrels, and raccoons also provided significant quantities. Gathering remained a valuable activity as well. Nuts, roots, wild fruits, and berries provided valuable calories and nutrients, especially during the relatively lean time between the end of the winter hunting season and the ripening of the first crops during the summer. A particular community occasionally relied upon another community for sustenance when one of its subsistence activities had poor results, but because little environmental variation existed with the Cherokees' homeland, the flow of food products from one town to the next was an exceptional case. Towns were arrayed in a linear fashion along a river that flowed out of the mountains, and each had equal access to the soil in the floodplain and wild game in upland forests. In normal times, horticulture, hunting, and gathering supplied each community with enough food for its residents to survive.[19]

Cherokees thus engaged in very little trade among their own villages and even much less with other groups. Each town had relatively the same access to lithic resources, firewood, salt, and other essential nonfood items and did not rely on gaining these from neighboring Cherokee communities much less from outside groups. To be sure some long-distance exchange in more exotic items and materials occurred. Southern Appalachian towns, for instance, acquired marine shell from the Atlantic and Gulf Coasts and copper from the Great Lakes region, while sending mica, deerskins, turkey feathers, and other things to outsiders.[20] Long-distance exchange, though, should not be inflated. Archaeologists have found that an overwhelming majority of grave goods in sites across the Southeast were made from local materials.[21] Nonlocal items, on the other hand, remained uncommon components of archaeological sites and were rarely transformed into utilitarian objects. Instead, exotic materials were made into status or ceremonial items, which often came to symbolize the power of leading individuals and families. Gorgets made of marine shell, headdresses adorned with images cut from sheet copper, and copper plates decorated with powerful cosmological symbols, for example, were included in several elite graves.[22] The presence of such goods, though, does not change the fact that exchange occurred at a low volume and at irregular intervals.[23]

Making aboriginal exchange even more irregular was the impact that warfare had on the social landscape in which Cherokees lived. Southeastern polities were more likely to fight than trade with each other. Scholars propose a variety of reasons why indigenous peoples warred with each other: communities used military action to acquire territory and control resources; young warriors depended on success in battle to gain status; families sought vengeance for the loss of their kinsmen; and leaders exercised force to defeat and humiliate their rivals as well as gain tribute from subordinate towns.[24] Whatever the cause of such conflict, years of endemic warfare created contested spaces or buffer zones between rival polities, where humans could not live, hunt, or travel safely. Buffer zones particularly existed in upland areas between rival polities inhabiting parallel river valleys. Such contested areas could also be found within river valleys themselves as polities often found themselves, warring with others either up- or downriver from them. At times conflict became so intense that vast areas of some river valleys, which held great horticultural potential, lay vacant. These areas consequently served as sanctuaries for wild game, which multiplied more rapidly in the relative absence of human predators.[25]

Buffer zones existed across the Southeast and particularly limited communication between Cherokees and their neighbors. Sometime before European contact, residents of the central Savannah Valley, for example, vacated their settlements and moved elsewhere, leaving an agriculturally valuable area for safer locations. Warring chiefdoms in the South Carolina and Georgia piedmont made it unsafe for the area to be resettled.[26] Endemic warfare also created buffer zones between the Cherokees and their neighbors to the west. Along the Tennessee, lower Little Tennessee, and lower Hiwassee Rivers, an assortment of towns could be found that in general had very different cultural traits from Cherokee villages found deeper in the mountains. Scholars largely believe these people to have been Muskogean-speaking peoples, who for reasons explained later in this chapter moved farther south and became part of the confederacy known to the English as "Creeks" in the late seventeenth century. At the time of European contact, several of these towns tended to be compactly settled and surrounded by palisades, a strong indication of their having hostile relations with Cherokees.[27] In general, it made more sense for Native communities to scatter their households along floodplains so that they could make more efficient use of soil, but times of war forced people to adopt less desirable settlement patterns. Cherokees, especially, had an ecological imperative to live in dispersed settlements as the river valleys they inhabited were fairly narrow and had more scattered patches of fertile soil, but even they resorted to fortified, compact villages to protect themselves from their multiple enemies.[28]

Given that they lived in simple chiefdoms, had limited connections to communities outside of southern Appalachia, and had buffer zones around them, one would expect Cherokees to be safe from exposure to a deadly germ introduced at a distant location. That Cherokees were an isolated exception among a North American population that smallpox destroyed, however, remains seriously doubtful. Even the larger chiefdoms of the Mississippi Valley should not strike anyone as particularly vulnerable to receiving smallpox from a distant location. These polities had much more in common with Cherokees than they did Aztecs and Incas. They were warring chiefdoms amid a maze of contested zones and were composed of economically redundant and self-sufficient communities, which engaged in limited long-distance trade. This trade certainly did not reach Mexico—to date no objects of Meso-American origin have been found in any southeastern archaeological site.[29] A hemispheric pandemic from Canada to Chile then is a story that metaphor and figurative language might convince people to believe but not a story that makes sense when one conducts a sober examination of the similarities and differences among Native societies of the Americas. For smallpox to arrive in the Southeast and particularly for it to reach southern Appalachia, European colonization had to have a more direct and significant impact on the region and its people.

• • • •

A direct introduction of *Variola* became a possibility in the sixteenth century with the intrusion of would-be European conquistadors, colonizers, and explorers. Before and during the immediate years of Saint Augustine's founding in 1565, the Spanish sponsored six major expeditions (Juan Ponce de León [1521]; Lucas Vázquez de Ayllón [1526]; Panfilo de Narváez [1528]; Hernando de Soto [1539–43]; Tristan de Luna [1559–61]; Juan Pardo [1566–68]), while the French sponsored one (Jean Ribault [1562–64]) that touched down at different places along the Atlantic or Gulf Coasts and stayed for varying lengths of time. For some scholars these fleeting contacts in what the Spanish called *La Florida* were enough to trigger epidemics that struck a myriad of Natives across the greater Southeast, even those who did not directly encounter any of the expeditions.[30]

Such conclusions, however, do not fit with basic epidemiology. If smallpox, for example, had accompanied any sixteenth-century expeditions, active cases among at least some members of the expedition would have been apparent between ten and fourteen days after departing their bases. These individuals then would have had either to come into direct contact with indigenous peoples within the virus's period of communicability or more likely had to have passed the disease onto other members of the expedition to keep a chain of infection going until the expedition contacted Natives. None of the accounts and chronicles of any of the sixteenth-century expeditions suggests any such infections occurred on board or shortly after coming ashore. To be sure, Europeans sickened and some died in the Southeast, but they did so from illnesses that began well after arriving, thus ruling out an acute infectious disease that must have necessarily begun to spread aboard their ships. Given the demographic makeup of sixteenth-century expeditions, this lack of transmission of smallpox makes sense. The majority of those who composed such adventures were adult males, a population that one would not suspect as being a viable conduit for the spread of *Variola*.[31] Smallpox and other acute infectious diseases in other words did not automatically spread in any contact situation. Still, there is one bit of evidence that proponents of the "virgin soil" thesis often cite to make a case that early exploration ignited epidemics. In 1540, the Hernando de Soto expedition made its way into the Carolina Piedmont and reached the central town of the Cofitachequi chiefdom. There, one of Soto's chroniclers reported, "About the town within the compass of a league and a half league were large uninhabited towns, choked with vegetation, which looked as though no people had inhabited them for some time." Natives informed the Spaniards that "two years ago there had been a plague in that land and they had moved to other towns."[32] A later and less reliable account of the Soto expedition called the disaster both a "pestilence" and a "plague" and mentioned four houses stacked with corpses.[33] The fact that Soto and his men found a metal dagger, rosary beads, and steel axes further supports the notion that a deadly colonial germ came with a fleeting contact experience between Natives and newcomers.[34]

It is indeed tempting to conclude that the "plague" of Cofitachequi was an outbreak of a novel disease, but scholars should be cautious in blaming newly introduced pathogens for Cofitachequi's fate. Soto's men did not directly observe the event; rather they learned of it from a Native interpreter, whose translation of the story into Spanish was certainly far from perfect and void of details. Europeans often used the terms plague and pestilence in generic ways to describe great sickness, and it is possible that the Spaniards misinterpreted the event as a plague when it was really a famine, an unfortunate but not uncommon phenomenon for southeastern horticulturalists. Floods, droughts, insect invasions, or a number of other problems could have destroyed harvests, resulting in widespread hunger and sickness due to common aboriginal diseases. In addition, the houses with piles of corpses need not be seen as evidence of catastrophic mortality from novel germs. Southeastern Natives commonly kept the bones of their ancestors in mortuary temples for veneration.[35] Soto's men, furthermore, may have been inclined to interpret the plague from perspectives shaped by earlier Spanish experiences. Many of them had participated in the conquests of the Aztecs, read about it, or heard about it and consequently knew about the devastation that smallpox had caused among natives in Mexico.

Assuming that the plague of Cofitachequi was a disease that Europeans introduced, what could it have been? The most likely culprit in this hypothetical situation was malaria. A chronic disease that persists within a human host for a fairly lengthy time, malaria could be spread from place to place with even fleeting contacts, assuming that carriers of *Plasmodia* arrived in an area in which *Anopheles* mosquitoes were present and did so during the warm season when the pests were active. Much of the North American continent, especially the American South, teemed with *Anopheles* prior to 1492, and it is not hard to imagine that sixteenth-century explorers stocked this animal reservoir with *Plasmodia*. In doing so, though, the newcomers did not ignite massive and widespread depopulation. Malaria's case fatality rate of 10 percent pales in comparison to smallpox's 40 percent and its impact would not have been evenly distributed. *Anopheles* mosquitos generally inhabit areas with swampy, slow-moving water with a viable mammal population on which to feed. Large agricultural societies along meandering rivers represented a highly vulnerable population to malaria, while smaller chiefdoms in highlands were less vulnerable. For those communities that came to suffer from this seasonal disease, disruption in agricultural production would also be expected as the cycle of fevers and chills typically peaked during harvest time. Conceivably, communities near Cofitachequi and those in other places in the Southeast particularly situated to sustain malaria abandoned their towns in the sixteenth century and did so after declining and perhaps even failed harvests. Not everyone in these particular towns perished. Instead, a majority survived and relocated to healthier places or did what de Soto's chroniclers reported: they moved to other towns that did not suffer the same circumstances.

• • • •

Rather than the ignition of epidemics, physical brutality against Natives proved to be the most significant legacy of early explorers of the

Southeast, especially as they ventured into southern Appalachia. In 1540 and 1567 respectively, Hernando de Soto's and Juan Pardo's expeditions crossed over the mountains just north of the Cherokees' historic homeland, and both encountered a diverse array of Native communities.[36] Some of these peoples were Iroquoian speakers and ancestral to the Cherokees, some were Muskogean speakers and ancestral to the Creeks, and some had identities that cannot be known. But, for the area's indigenous population in general, encounters with the Spanish provided a harsh introduction to the violent era of colonization.

Using a combination of archaeological, linguistic, and documentary evidence, scholars have recently made great strides identifying several chiefdoms that the Spaniards visited as ancestral to the more familiar indigenous nations of the eighteenth century.[37] Such evidence ironically rules out one province that the Spanish traveled through as having a direct link to the Cherokee Nation.[38] Soto came upon "Chalaque" east of the Appalachians and learned of its name from his Muskogean-speaking interpreter in whose language Chalaque meant "people who spoke a different language."[39] The name at that time applied to Siouan speakers, who ultimately coalesced into the Catawba Nation.[40] The English, of course, later gave the epithet of Muskogean origin greater currency and applied it to Iroquoian speakers in the mountains, although rendering it into the more well-known "Cherokee" by making the common substitution of a hard "r" for a soft "l." The Spaniards began to meet people who likely spoke an Iroquoian language as they moved up the Catawba River and over the mountains. Both Soto and Pardo entered "Joara" at the headwaters of the Catawba River, while Pardo veered off his predecessor's path and visited "Tanasqui" on the Nolichucky River and "Tocae" on the French Broad.[41] All three towns appear equivalent to towns commonly spelled as Jore, Tanasi, and Toqua—towns that belonged to the eighteenth-century Cherokees, although in locations farther to the south and west than where Pardo visited them.[42] On the Pigeon River, Pardo entered "Cauchi," which does not have a clear equivalent in later records but which archaeologists believe to be the Garden Creek site, a place where Cherokee material culture prevailed.[43] In his journey across the mountains, Pardo also met representatives that travelled from "Xenaca," "Neguase," "Estate," "Tacuru," "Utaca," and "Quetua."[44] These names all appear equivalent to important eighteenth-century Cherokee towns commonly spelled as Seneca, Nikwasi, Estatoe, Tugaloo, Watagi, and Kituwha.[45] One other group might have been ancestral to the Cherokee Nation. The Spanish located the Chisca chiefdom in southwestern Virginia, a place where archaeologists have identified some Cherokee material culture but have not made even a tentative conclusion about the chiefdom's association with an eighteenth-century nation.[46]

Spanish accounts then provide evidence that at least some sixteenth-century Cherokees resided in settlements north and east of their later location. Oral history supports this conclusion. Catawbas claimed Cherokees once resided in the upper reaches of the Catawba Valley, an area where the Spanish found Joara, but a long and bitter war between the two Native groups led the latter to abandon the area and move west.[47] Eighteenth-century Cherokees recalled that some of the constituents of the Overhill Towns once lived along the Noli-chucky, where Pardo visited Tanasqui, while nineteenth-century Cherokees remembered that the Middle Settlements received an influx of people from the French Broad, where the Spanish found Tocae.[48] That their ancestors had once lived where the Spanish located Chiscas also figures prominently in Cherokee oral history. In 1809, Selukuki Wohellengh, a noted chief and speaker, remarked that the "earliest traditions say that our ancestors inhabited near the heads of this river: (the Tennessee or its branches of Holston)."[49] In 1826, Charles Hicks, a bilingual Cherokee who served as a chief and official interpreter of his nation, echoed Selukuki Wohellengh. Hicks claimed that his ancestors traveled from where the sun rises but rested in the lands between the Clinch, Holston, and Cumberland Rivers before coming to reside in their historic location.[50] Hicks did not provide details about when and why his ancestors moved south and west, but such a journey appears to have been common knowledge within his nation.[51] Whether any of these groups were the Chiscas remains conjectural of course, but Native oral history as a whole corresponds well with what documentary, linguistic, and archaeological evidence tell us:

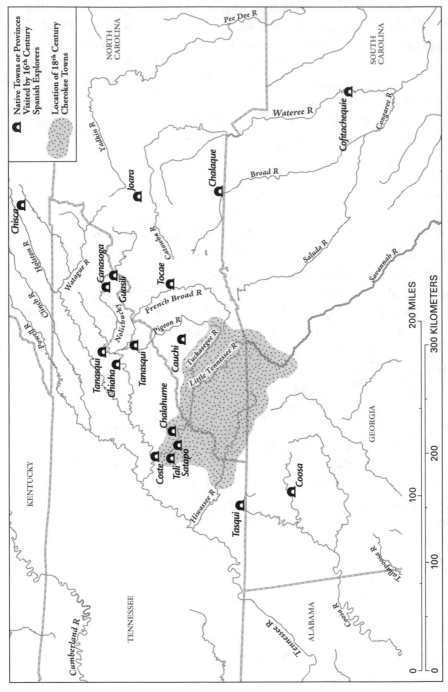

Soto (1540) and Pardo (1567–68) expeditions. Map by Darin Grauberger and Meghan Kelly, University of Kansas Cartographic Services.

some sixteenth-century Cherokees lived outside of their historic homeland and later relocated farther to the south and west after de Soto's
and Pardo's intrusions.

The same multiplicity of evidence indicates that the peoples the
Spanish visited in what is today eastern Tennessee were not ancestors to the Cherokees, even though they resided where the Overhill
Towns existed in the eighteenth century. The Spanish identified
several native towns, including Chiaha, Coste, Tali, Satapo, Chala-
hume, and Tasqui, whose names appear to be Muskogean in origin.
Chiaha, Coste, and Tasqui show up over a century later in a more
southern location and as part of the Muskogee or Creek Confederacy.[52]
The archaeological record furthermore reveals marked differences
between peoples who lived in eastern Tennessee and Iroquoian
speakers deeper in the mountains. Sometime after the Spanish visited
an abrupt cultural change occurred. Settlement patterns, housing
styles, and ceramic patterns changed considerably, indicating that a
new people came in and displaced the area's residents.[53] Oral history
augments this interpretation. In the early nineteenth century, John
Norton, a literate Mohawk of Cherokee ancestry, visited his relatives
and recorded them as saying "that when they came from the northeast, they drove the Creeks, or Muscogue, from the country bordering
on the Tennessee." One village of Muskogees in particular existed
on an island at the junction of the Ocoee and Hiwassee. Norton saw
for himself mounds and "ancient corn fields" that confirmed Cherokee claims.[54] Of course, these original Muskogean dwellers, who had
encountered Soto's expedition, did not necessarily all move from
the region. It is possible that some became engulfed by Iroquoian
speakers at some point and assimilated with Cherokees. In any event,
a significant demographic change occurred in eastern Tennessee after
Soto explored the area. Most if not all Muskogean speakers moved
out, Iroquoians moved in, and in the process the Overhill division
of the Cherokee Nation emerged.

The Spanish, to be sure, may have played no part in the demographic transitions that occurred in southern Appalachia. English-
sponsored slave raids, which will be discussed later in this chapter,
certainly caused a movement of Cherokees south and west and flight
of some groups from the mountains. Spanish brutality, nevertheless,

cannot be ruled out as a contributing factor. Soto, an officer who participated in Pizarro's conquest of the Incas, advanced through the Southeast with a ruthlessness that Natives had never seen before. Today, it appears remarkable that some six hundred Spanish soldiers could have made their way across the Southeast without being wiped out by the much more numerous Natives. But, two things must be kept in mind. First, most Native societies that Soto encountered were simple chiefdoms that would have found it difficult to mobilize as many as six hundred fighters. Second, the Spanish possessed superior military technology. Firearms gave some advantage. Soto's men carried a few arquebuses—primitive guns with little accuracy but whose loud noise and smoke certainly terrorized Natives. Soto's men also wore metal armor that could deflect stone tipped arrows and used metal swords that could easily slash through wooden and leather shields. Horses, most of all, gave the Spanish an advantage. Natives had never seen these beasts before, making a well-organized cavalry charge of armored and sword-wielding soldiers nearly impossible to stop.[55] Soto employed such superiority to steal food for his army and its horses, imprison leaders and hold them for ransom, and enslave individuals and force them to serve as porters in his arduous track. Wherever Soto's army went it left a trail of destruction.

Their route across the mountains and down the western side of the Appalachians was no exception. Soto and his men demanded and took food during the early growing season when Natives regularly experienced a period of want.[56] At Chiaha, for example, Soto found an obstinate people and punished them by destroying their "large maize fields."[57] Soto's rampage continued as he moved south. At Coste his foot soldiers found no food in obvious sight and pillaged each house, taking what they could find.[58] When some Natives violently objected, Soto had the leader and some of his principal men put into chains, telling them "that he would burn all of them, because they had laid hands on the Christians."[59] At Coosa, the Spaniards again rested for a few weeks, holding the leader hostage and helping themselves to the food surpluses stored at the center of this important chiefdom. Upon his departure, Soto "seized many . . . men and women" and put them in chains. Each Spanish man "took away as slaves those he had in chains, without allowing them to go to their lands."[60]

Pardo caused harm as well—especially to Chisca, a province that the Spanish thought possessed gold. In January 1567, the Spanish captain had a small outpost built and christened Fort San Juan near the town of Joara. Thirty soldiers garrisoned the outpost and consequently altered interchiefdom relations in the area. Under the command of Sgt. Hernando Moyano, fifteen Spaniards and an untold number of indigenous auxiliaries from Joara ventured out to punish Chisca's leader who refused to welcome the Spanish. The sergeant reported that his forces killed one thousand Natives and burned fifty houses. The leader of Chisca apparently did not back down and sent a threatening message to Moyano and his men, claiming "he would come and eat them and a dog that the sergeant had." The sergeant's second attack, though, inflicted terrible damage. The Spanish managed to breach the defenses of a "well fortified" town, slaughter all that they could find, and set all of its dwellings ablaze, killing 1,500 Natives in the process.[61] Spanish accounts may have certainly exaggerated the numbers killed in Chisca, but they nonetheless reveal that Europeans intervened in a rivalry between Native polities and inflicted severe damage. Pardo's forces may have in fact been responsible for the collapse of the Chisca chiefdom and flight of its people from southwest Virginia, something that certainly happened before English goods arrived in the area.[62] The Spanish meanwhile did not ingratiate themselves too well with their supposed allies. By May 1568, Natives sacked and burned Fort San Juan and other outposts that Pardo had left in the interior.[63]

One need not imagine that either Soto or Pardo introduced lethal microbes to produce demographic changes in southern Appalachia. Neither expedition carried any novel germ more dangerous than malaria, and the impact of this disease would have been eclipsed by the Spaniards' violence and theft of vital food supplies. It is possible that exploration parties in fact led to at least some areas of southern Appalachia being depopulated. Perhaps the trauma that they inflicted started the process of Native residents leaving the upper Tennessee drainage, including the Holston, Clinch, Powell, Nolichucky, and French Broad and coalescing farther south with towns that were already there and in the process adding to the Lower, Middle, and Valley divisions of the Cherokee Nation. Cherokee oral history suggests such an occurrence and indicates a subsequent movement farther into eastern Tennessee. Perhaps Spanish exploration in this region destabilized and weakened the Muskogean chiefdoms in that area and facilitated the expansion of Iroquoian-speaking peoples into what became known as the Overhill Towns of the Cherokee Nation. These demographic changes, if they indeed began in the mid-sixteenth century, were nonetheless not exclusively the result of the Spaniard's brutality. As we will see later, the English during the last half of the seventeenth century sponsored a trade in Native slaves, an activity that reoriented indigenous societies toward the Atlantic world and produced a shatter zone of violence, disease, and depopulation.

• • • •

After Pardo's departure, no known European presence in southern Appalachia occurred until the late seventeenth century. Still, the possibility existed that an epidemic erupting somewhere else on the North American continent could have spread to Cherokees. Recorded outbreaks certainly occurred in Florida among Natives in close association with the Spanish and in the Northeast among indigenous peoples in close contact with the English, Dutch, and French who settled there. Did the influence of these distant European colonies extend into southern Appalachia and link the Cherokees' ancestors into a chain of infection?

Let us start with the Spanish. In 1565, the Spanish founded Saint Augustine—the first permanent European settlement in what becomes the United States—and immediately sponsored the missionary activities of Catholic priests, who fanned out along the Atlantic Coast and Florida panhandle. By 1639, their missions stretched northward to near the Savannah River and westward to the Apalachicola River. Thousands of Timucuas, Guales, and Apalachees lived in the missions, which not only served as centers for religious conversion but also units of production in the larger Spanish Empire. Native converts supplied the Spanish with food and labor, and they made frequent trips along the trails and paths that linked their villages to Saint Augustine. Ultimately, new diseases were introduced to Spanish Florida and radiated out from Saint Augustine to the various missions. In 1617, for example, Franciscan priests remarked that "great plagues [*pestes*] and contagious sicknesses" had struck their missions over the past four years, leaving over half of the Timucua and Guale converts in their graves.[64] A "plague" of an unknown disease struck Saint Augustine in 1649, and then in 1657 the Spanish recorded a smallpox epidemic for the first time in their colony.[65] By 1680, the indigenous population had plummeted dramatically. One scholar estimates that by that year, 90 percent of the Timucua population had disappeared.[66]

That any of the epidemics that ravaged Spanish Florida in the seventeenth century made their way into southern Appalachia remains conjectural at best. Smallpox and other diseases reached converted communities because they had been integrated into a larger flow of tribute and goods that circulated throughout the Spanish Empire. Missionaries and colonial officials facilitated an unprecedented flow of people and goods across old contested areas that had formerly separated the Apalachees, Timucuas, and Guales. Spanish colonialism, however, had little impact outside of the mission system. Trade disseminating from Florida remained minimal. Hostility generally characterized the relationship between those in the mission communities and their immediate neighbors, thus creating buffer zones across which diseases would have had a difficult time traveling. The Spanish in fact frowned upon any activities other than proselytizing. Trade outside of the missions was prohibited, and while it still occurred clandestinely, it did so at a low volume. Few converted Natives proved willing to serve as guides or porters carrying goods to their enemies to the north.[67] Spanish goods did occasionally make it out of Florida but likely did so through low-volume down-the-line trading or through sporadic raiding on mission communities rather than a high volume of sustained trading, such as what the English would initiate during the latter half of the seventeenth century. Spanish goods that show up in the archaeological record outside of Florida indeed are few in number in comparison to the amount of English trade goods that have been discovered among the remains of colonial era indigenous communities in the Southeast.[68] It thus remains doubtful that smallpox or any other of the Atlantic world's deadliest germs escaped Florida's indigenous populations, made their way across buffer zones, and infected the myriad of Native communities that had yet to be transformed by colonialism.

For similar reasons, *Variola*'s arrival in southern Appalachia from the north seems improbable. Major epidemics occurred among the Iroquois in the 1630s and 1660s and possibly spread by way of their captive raids.[69] Still, two factors suggest that the virus remained to the north. First, there is a paucity of references to smallpox in colonial Virginia. One would think that had smallpox descended from the north and had it reached as far south as the Cherokees' homeland that the disease would have also struck some of the tribes known to the Virginians and would have spawned some written accounts. The only documented instance of smallpox striking Natives within or near the Virginia colony that existed before the 1690s occurred in 1667, when infected sailors passed it on to a small tribe residing on the Eastern Shore.[70] The outbreak did not spread beyond that location.[71] Second, Iroquois raiding activities against southern tribes appear to have been minimal before 1701. For most of the seventeenth century, the Iroquois had their hands full with French-allied tribes to their north and west. Those tribes bore the brunt of Iroquois attacks and consequently fell victim to smallpox epidemics that ravaged the Five Nations. The Great Peace of 1701, mediated in part by the French that quelled conflict between the Five Nations and the numerous groups in Canada and around the Great Lakes, redirected Iroquois warfare activities to the South.[72] By then, however, English traders out of Virginia and South Carolina had already integrated the Cherokees into a trade network that served as a more viable avenue for smallpox to take.

• • • •

English commerce, especially in Native slaves, served as the most likely mechanism to ignite an epidemic among Cherokees that went unrecorded. Beginning in Virginia around 1660 and then escalating after South Carolina's founding in 1670, English traders trucked guns, ammunition, alcohol, and other desirable goods to Natives in return for the prisoners that they took in war. This trade radically transformed the Southeast and its indigenous population. It substantially increased the level of violence, as gun-wielding groups traveled far and wide in search for prisoners that they could trade to the English. Before this commerce collapsed with the Yamasee War (1715–18), tens of thousands of Natives had been enslaved to white masters in Virginia and South Carolina or shipped to the slave markets of the West Indies. Thousands had died in the violence associated with raiding, while thousands more had been made refugees, fleeing their homes in the wake of raids and huddling behind palisade walls of compact defensive towns. The slave trade had been truly transformative, bringing colonialism fully into a region that had been marginal to European expansion.[73]

The English built the Native slave trade on aboriginal practices of captive taking. By returning to their communities with enemies taken alive, male warriors gained considerable status. Captors might have ritually tortured and killed their prisoners, especially males, to avenge the loss of kinsmen killed in battle, or they might have chosen to adopt captives, especially women and children, to replace deceased loved ones.[74] When the English offered a variety of new and useful goods for these slaves, indigenous peoples did not completely abandon their traditional ways in which they dealt with prisoners, but the lure of such items was great, leading to an escalation of warfare and a high number of captives falling into the possession of Europeans. The preponderance of women and children taken also increased. English masters especially wanted to buy young boys and girls as well as older females. Native men proved especially troublesome slaves, since they came from societies in which they did not perform agricultural field work. Male captives who remained enslaved on plantations in Virginia and Carolina also had high rates of flight. Native raiders acquiesced to the demands of their English partners by purposely attacking their enemies to gain particular types of captives. Of course, this in part reflects Native desires as well, since they wanted to keep male warriors for ritual torture to fulfill cultural obligations to their deceased kinsmen. Nevertheless, the desire for English trade goods led indigenous raiders to seize females and children in far greater numbers than they had been doing before contact.[75]

Native captors found immense rewards for the fruits of their labors. Woolen clothing, which remained relatively soft even after becoming wet and drying, offered more comfort than buckskins, which when dried out became stiff, cracked, and irritating to the wearer; metal pots did not break when dropped and could be reshaped into sheet brass and cut into arrowheads; and iron hatchets spared Native artisans of the difficult task of chipping hard stones to form tools needed on an everyday basis. Natives also came to desire another trade item, alcohol, which had no material value but which was quickly consumed and created a desire for more. European colonial authorities frequently attempted to regulate the distribution of rum, brandy, and other intoxicating beverages, but alcohol flowed into indigenous villages despite official prohibitions. At times, liquor came sporadically, and at other times, when officials relaxed regulations or even actively encouraged its distribution, it flooded into Native communities, leading to more warring, slaving, and hunting to supply the English with the goods they so eagerly sought.[76] The commodity, however, that had the most profound impact on indigenous peoples was the gun. As with alcohol, firearms created the need for further trade. A gun in itself was useless without a constant supply of powder and shot, and its adoption as a weapon of choice required continuous relations with European suppliers.

Cherokees probably first felt the impact of the Native slave trade in the 1650s as victims of raids. Virginians formed an alliance with the Westoes, who moved south and established themselves near the Fall Line of the Savannah River by 1659. They warred against a number of enemies, possibly the Cherokees who lived not far away but certainly peoples within the Spanish missions of Florida.[77] At the same time, Virginia's leading traders were sending out caravans loaded with manufactured goods on a path that led southwesterly to Siouan-speaking groups just to the east of the Blue Ridge.[78] Catawbas, the descendants of these groups, in fact recalled that they came to possess firearms before Cherokees and used this advantage to drive their neighbors deeper into the mountains.[79] Another armed group who attacked Cherokee towns was the Tomahitans, a tribe whose ethnic affiliation remains unclear. Since at least 1673, the Tomahitans had been trading with Siouan middlemen. They lived deep in the Appalachian Mountains, possessed sixty guns, waged war on enemies both far and near, and in the process acquired numerous

child captives. Such violence shattered southern Appalachian communities and led to an exodus of at least some peoples from the
mountains.[80] One refugee group from southern Appalachia became
part of the Yamasees, a diverse collection of people that fled into
Florida in the 1680s. Cherokees later referred to them as their "ancient
people" and remembered them as being driven away by the Tomahitans.[81] What happened to the Tomahitans themselves remains unclear.
They may have become a part of the Cherokee Nation, whose roster of
towns in the eighteenth century included a Tomatly, or they may have
been driven out in whole or in part from the highlands. The English
trader James Adair, for example, listed the "Ta-me-tah" as a refugee
group that fled from the north and confederated with the Creeks.[82]

Regardless of the Tomahitans final destiny, Cherokees ultimately
became Virginia's partners. Following Bacon's Rebellion in 1676—a
war in which Virginians attacked and drove away a variety of Native
peoples from the frontiers of their colony, English traders had more
direct access to southern Appalachia.[83] The Siouan towns, which
had controlled the southwesterly flow of goods, had been dealt a
severe blow and were forced along with a number of other groups
to flee farther south. William Byrd I (1652–1704) was certainly one
of those traders who cashed in on new trading opportunities. Byrd,
the patriarch of one of early America's most famous families, gained
much of his wealth and status through trading with Natives. His son,
William II, later remarked that his father had been one of the first
Englishmen to trade with Cherokees.[84] Another leading Virginian,
Cadwallader Jones, also capitalized on an open route to southern
Appalachia. By 1682, he was sending out his packhorse caravans from
Virginia on a southwestern course of four hundred miles.[85]

Once incorporated into Virginia's trade network, Cherokees turned
from victims to victimizers in the Native slave trade. As early as 1681,
the Spanish recorded the "Chalaque" among several armed groups
that raided Catholic missions for slaves.[86] Five years later, the Spanish
learned that several groups had fled from the north, escaping from
the "Chalaque" and other English-allied groups. Among those who
fled were the Koasati that ultimately became part of the Creek Confederacy.[87] That these "Chalaque" were Cherokees is supported by
oral history previously discussed in this chapter, which holds that

they expanded into eastern Tennessee at the expense of the Creeks whom they displaced. The movement of Iroquoian-speaking people into eastern Tennessee may have started back in the sixteenth century after Spanish exploration destabilized chiefdoms in the area, but the bulk of the evidence suggest that this process was not complete by the 1680s. Then, armed Iroquoian speakers displaced or absorbed gunless Muskogean speakers and in the process established the Overhill Towns.

Cherokees did not benefit from their alliance with Virginia very long before South Carolina made them victims again of English colonialism. South Carolina greatly expanded the volume of exchange involving human captives and guns. Cherokees first show up in Carolinian records in 1674, when Henry Woodward traveled to the Savannah River, where he learned that the "Chorakees" lived on the river's branches.[88] In 1681, a similar sounding name appears in South Carolina's records. Then, the English exported several "Seraquii" slaves.[89] In 1690, at least one Carolinian played a direct role in conducting raids on the Cherokees. James Moore, an ambitious slave trader who fantasized that southern Appalachia contained gold and silver, twice ventured into the mountains to seek his fortune. Moore claimed that "a difference about trade" caused the mountain Natives to turn him back, but Carolina's proprietors learned that his search for wealth turned into a homicidal raid, exclaiming: "Without any war first proclaimed, [Moore had] fallen upon the Cherokee Indians in a hostile manner and murdered several of them."[90] Three years later, Carolina's indigenous partners did even more damage. Shawnees and Yuchis, the Commons House of Assembly learned, "had been at one of the [Cherokee's] towns and meeting only with ye old men there (the young men being absent) killed them and carried away the women and children and sold some of them . . . to the English traders who had brought them to this settlement and sold them for slaves."[91] In the same year, several Cherokee chiefs traveled to Charles Town to complain about the treatment that Carolina's partners had inflicted upon them.[92] They condemned the Shawnees as well as two Siouan groups the Esaws and the Congarees, who together had destroyed several Cherokee towns and sold their people into slavery.

Carolinian officials told the Cherokees that their people had already been shipped off and nothing could be done.[93]

• • • •

By the late 1690s, then, the Cherokee world had undergone dramatic changes. They had been incorporated into larger trading networks that directly linked them not only to European colonies but also to a larger Atlantic world in which captives, guns, and goods flowed in relatively high volumes. At the same time the level and type of violence escalated around them and produced demographic changes that need not be associated with the arrival of smallpox. But, was smallpox also involved in shattering the Cherokees' world? Did the Cherokees' world change enough to facilitate the spread of colonialism's most dreaded germ to their southern Appalachian villages?

That smallpox arrived in the Southeast in the late 1690s is beyond doubt. Europeans in many parts of the Southeast left a vivid record of the germ as it seized the opportunity that the Native slave trade provided. This outbreak—the Great Southeastern Smallpox Epidemic—began in Virginia in 1696 and then proceeded southward down the coast and into the Carolina Piedmont.[94] Richard Traunter, a trader from the Old Dominion, stumbled upon a Siouan group in the throes of the epidemic and remarked: "These Indians received me kindly, though at that time they were very much dejected for the loss of their friends and relations, the smallpox having been brought amongst them which distemper they never knew before, and was the cause of their mortality and hardly a person in the nation escaped this distemper, whereof some hundred dyed."[95] The virus soon thereafter made it to South Carolina and then traveled to a variety of indigenous groups. "The smallpox hath killed so many [Natives]," South Carolinian officials reported in 1698, "that we have little reason to believe they will be capable of doing any harm to us for several years to come, that distemper having swept off great numbers of them 4 or 500 miles inland as well upon the seacoast as in our neighborhood."[96] Natives indeed suffered terribly as one English colonist described: "The whole country is full of trouble & sickness, tis the smallpox which has been mortal to all sorts of the inhabitants & especially the Indians who tis said to have swept away a whole neighboring nation, all to 5 or 6 which ran away and left their dead unburied, lying upon the ground for the vultures to devour."[97]

Slaving activities propelled the virus across a vast geographic expanse. It made its way along the trading paths that connected Carolina to its Muskogean partners located in present-day Georgia, Alabama, and Mississippi and then proceeded to the Gulf Coast, where it struck victims of captive raids. In 1699, for example, Pierre Le Moyne sieur d'Iberville explored Mobile Bay looking for a place to establish the new colony of Louisiana and found such "a prodigious number of human skeletons that they formed a mountain."[98] The French officer came to believe that they had died in a massacre but his countrymen later learned that the corpses were those of "a numerous nation who being pursued and having withdrawn to this region, had almost all died here of sickness."[99] Those pursuing these unfortunate people were certainly English-allied slave raiders, while the culprit that made them sick was smallpox. To the west of Mobile, Le Moyne d'Iberville came upon the Mougoulachas and Bayogoulas united in a single village and found a ghastly scene. Le Moyne d'Iberville reported that "the smallpox, which they still had in the village, had killed one-fourth of the people." The Natives placed these newly dead victims on scaffolds outside their village, making a wretched smell that made the French sick.[100] The French also found Native refugees in the Mississippi Valley, where they huddled in fortified settlements, fearing English-sponsored slave raids and tragically suffering mass mortality.[101]

Despite the numerous written accounts of the epidemic, no European actually referred specifically to Cherokees as victims.[102] There are good reasons to suspect, however, that the late 1690s marks the beginning of the Cherokees' experience with the most dangerous of colonial germs. They had been trading with Virginians, whose colony served as the launching pad for the disease to spread widely by way of traders, Native middlemen, captives, and runaway slaves. By 1698, the virus certainly made it to the Cherokees' most immediate neighbor to the east, the Catawbas, leading one to think that smallpox had a high probability of reaching at least those Cherokee settlements

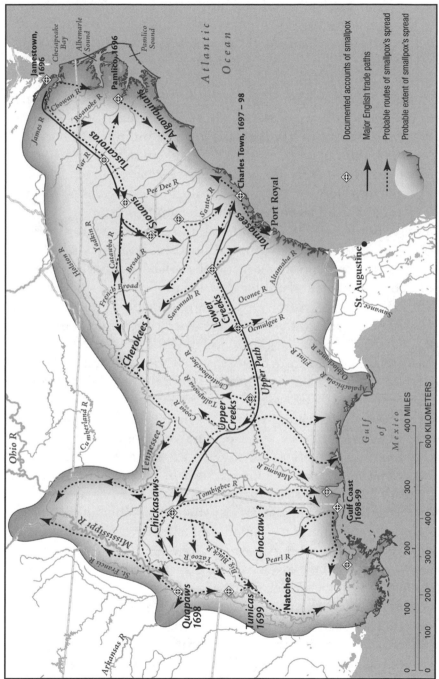

The Great Southeastern Smallpox Epidemic, 1696–1700. Map by Darin Grauberger and Meghan Kelly, University of Kansas Cartographic Services.

closest to Virginia. The dreaded scourge also could have reached southern Appalachia by way of South Carolina. Cherokees may have been buffered somewhat from the epidemic because their relationship with Carolina involved more enmity than friendship. Yet, as victims of raids, they stood a chance of becoming infected by those who sought to capture them or by their people escaping back to their home villages after being enslaved. Other victimized groups across the Southeast appear to have become infected through just such a process. As victims of raids, moreover, Cherokees must have had no choice but to live in defensive and compact villages, which forced their people into close living arrangements in which disease, once it arrived, could spread more easily from person to person.

Details about the 1738–39 epidemic in fact indicate an earlier exposure that could have happened forty years prior. Cherokee experience with smallpox in the late 1730s will be discussed in more detail in the next chapter, but for now, some clues from this documented epidemic are instructive in dating smallpox's first arrival. James Adair commented that "young married couples" suffered the most, a statement that suggests individuals who had reached middle age were relatively safe from the disease.[103] Thomas Eyre, an official from the new colony of Georgia backed up Adair's comment stating that Cherokees had lost "most of their young men" to the disease.[104] A sizable portion of the indigenous nation in other words appears to have acquired immunity sometime before 1738. Population estimates that the English made offer further evidence. Adair commented off handedly that smallpox took "almost one half" of the Cherokees, but his estimate appears to be exaggerated. Georgians who actually spoke to Cherokees in the immediate aftermath of the epidemic reported a loss of one thousand of the nation's total five thousand warriors, which meant that the entire population likely shrank by a somewhat smaller percentage if the disease took a disproportionate number of young men.[105] South Carolina's officials did not share the view that Cherokees numbered some 5,000 warriors before the epidemic; their most recent count taken in 1721 put the number of warriors at 3,510.[106] But the colony's governor adjusted Cherokee strength downward by about the same percentage that the Georgians did. In 1742, Gov. William Bull reported the number of Cherokee warriors at an even

3,000, which would mean a 15 percent population loss.[107] Both Georgia's and South Carolina's postepidemic figures were inexact, but at the very least they convey a perception of the 1738–39 epidemic as severe but not as severe as a first exposure would have been. On one hand, a 15 percent to 20 percent loss was certainly devastating, especially when most of these deceased were young people of reproductive age. The epidemic in other words exacted long-term demographic damage on the entire nation. On the other hand, the numbers do not approach the 40 percent mortality rate that one might expect with a first experience with smallpox. There almost certainly had to be a prior exposure, and, given that people who had reached middle age fared comparatively well in the late 1730s, this earlier and first exposure most likely happened thirty to forty years earlier.

Cherokee oral history, although with some ambiguity, gives support for smallpox's arrival in the late 1690s. In narrating Cherokee history, Charles Hicks referred to a devastating epidemic sometime before a particular war broke out with the Creeks: "It must have been before this war had took place when the smallpox had been introduced in the nation by some visitant Cherokees from the seashore, which became so destructive to the inhabitants of the Valley Towns in depopulating mostly whole towns; and in some whole families falling victims to this epidemic's disorder, and only two towns had escaped from this epidemic destroyer." If the war in question was the Yamasee War (1715–18), then the epidemic either occurred in the 1690s or 1710s. Hicks added that smallpox arrived at about the same time as did Cornelius Doherty, whom the Cherokees remembered as the first white trader to introduce European goods. Based on details that Hicks learned about Doherty's life—that he came into their nation at the age of 30 and lived among them until 1779 when he died at the age of 111—the devastating epidemic occurred exactly in 1698![108] Such a conclusion of course remains problematic due to Doherty's improbable age at death and the fact that another source put the English trader's arrival in the year 1719.[109] Hicks, however, may have been conflating a series of major events—the arrival of English traders, who certainly worked if not lived among Cherokees by the late 1690s, a war with the Creeks that began around 1715, and the introduction of smallpox which happened somewhere in between. His account thus should not be rejected out of hand. His grim description and his placement of the event in 1698 matches exactly what European documents verify in fact happened among so many nearby Natives at the time.

• • • •

To be sure, one cannot rule out an even later first arrival of *Variola* among Cherokees, perhaps in 1711 or in 1718 when the disease returned to Charles Town. During these years, English trade continued to extend into southern Appalachia and even more so than during the 1690s. Germs had the potential to hitch a ride with the human traffic that went back and forth from the coast to the highlands. As in the 1690s, no documents exist that explicitly identify Cherokees as victims of either smallpox outbreak. But this time the absences are more telling. By the 1710s, Cherokees had emerged as South Carolina's most important Native trading partner and military ally. The indigenous nation figured prominently into the colony's written records, and one would think if smallpox made its inaugural impact in either 1711 or 1718 then English officials would have taken note of it.

In the early 1700s, South Carolina became more aggressive in building its relationship with Cherokees. Virginia had dominated the Cherokee trade, but Carolinians concluded that the Cherokees as well as the Catawbas fell into their dominion. In 1707, Carolinian officials confiscated the goods of Virginians and shut down the flow of trade from the Old Dominion for nearly a decade. South Carolinians rushed into the vacuum. "The [Cherokee] nation now entirely subject to us," one colonial agent wrote "are extremely well [situated] to keep off any incursions which . . . French Indians may think of making into Carolina and in effect so it is, they are now our only defense."[110] By 1710, Carolinian traders made regular trips from Charles Town, escorting trains of packhorses loaded with goods that had been in short supply among the Cherokees, while returning to the colonial capital with deerskins and slaves.[111] Not surprisingly then the English called upon Cherokees for assistance during the Tuscarora War (1711–13). The Tuscaroras lived near the Atlantic Coast of North Carolina and had attempted to expel settlers who encroached upon their

homeland, but in doing so they drew the attention of South Carolina's leading men and slave dealers. In 1712, Col. John Barnwell
led an attempt to reduce the Tuscaroras to submission, but after
forcing them to sign a treaty and enslaving nearly two hundred, the
Natives resumed their resistance. In 1713, Col. James Moore, Jr.,
returned to deliver the fatal blow and this time Carolinians had 310
Cherokee warriors to assist. Moore's forces killed or captured over
900 Tuscaroras and forced survivors to become either tributary groups
to the English colonies or flee to New York and join the Iroquois
Confederacy. An untold number of the captives wound up in Cherokee hands.[112] Cherokees had arrived as the major Native force near
Great Britain's southern colonies.

At the same time as the Tuscarora War, another round of smallpox
struck South Carolina. English colonists widely reported its presence
in and around Charles Town from May 1711 into spring 1712.[113] The
outbreak certainly struck some Native communities, but European
observers simply referred to "Indians" in general rather than giving
specific group names. In November 1711, for example, the Anglican
missionary Gideon Johnston exclaimed, "Never was there a more
sickly or fatal season than this, for the smallpox, pestilential fevers,
pleurisies, and fluxes have destroyed great numbers here of all sorts,
. . . whites, blacks, and Indians—and these distempers still rage to
an uncommon degree."[114] While one wishes that Johnston had been
more specific when referring to the epidemic, it is not hard to understand why the disease's impact among Natives did not receive the
detailed notice that it did in the 1690s. Then, the disease found numerous communities in which all their residents had no acquired immunity and exploded into a massive epidemic, but as a result, it left a
portion of the surviving indigenous population immunized. When
the virus returned, it circulated among the few nonimmunes, igniting
smaller, less noticeable outbreaks. These outbreaks, to be sure, had
serious consequences as the virus found most of its victims in the
preteen age group, thus making it even more difficult for Native
groups to recover from the Great Southeastern Smallpox Epidemic.
Given the Cherokees growing relationship with South Carolina, it
is not unimaginable that smallpox reached them as well either in 1711
or 1712. Nevertheless, the English made no record of it—suggesting

either the germ never reached them or that it did but caused minimal losses among a population with the majority of individuals having recently acquired immunity.

Variola again posed a threat to Cherokees at the end of the Yamasee War (1715–18). The Great Southeastern Smallpox Epidemic and a series of outbreaks of other diseases played an important role in the origins of this multitribal effort to destroy the settlers of South Carolina. English-allied groups had trouble finding enough captives to supply their trading partners and had a different idea of what would become of the captives that they did acquire: they would be adopted as kinsmen to make up for their own lost population. The Yamasees, who had eventually settled around Port Royal and became active participants in Carolina's slave raids, in particular lost more than 50 percent of their populations between 1696 and 1715 and could no longer afford to surrender their captives to pay off debts they owed to Carolinians. Traders, however, who had debts of their own to pay off, resorted to stealing captives, even those that had been adopted, and in doing so sowed the seeds for a revolt. The Lower Creeks too suffered terrible losses and deeply resented English traders stealing their adopted people. After coming to believe that all of South Carolina's allies would join them, the Yamasees and Lower Creeks initiated the revolt on April 15, 1715, when they executed Carolinian officials then visiting them. Within a matter of days, Carolinian traders throughout the Southeast were murdered. Warriors from multiple groups launched raids against outlying English settlements and caused Charles Town to swell with refugees. The colony that had done so much to spark the deadly cycle of slave raids and epidemics that brought its own allies on the brink of demographic collapse was now on the verge of its own demise.[115]

At the beginning of the war, Cherokees fought against South Carolina. Two factors explain their choice to do so. First, they had always had a connection to the Yamasees, a group whose constituents included former residents of southern Appalachia.[116] Second, Cherokees had their own grievances against the colonists in South Carolina. Since the 1680s, Carolinian slave dealers had purchased Cherokee captives, a practice that still continued in the eighteenth century. In 1706, for example, a group of traders engineered a brief war between Cherokees and Upper Creeks and then profited from the conflict by buying captives from each nation and then sending them into English settlements. Several Cherokees, at least those not shipped off to West Indian slave markets, suffered imprisonment on nearby plantations.[117] Suspicions of South Carolina's malevolent intentions were further heightened by a renegade trader who supposedly informed Cherokees that the "English [were] going to make wars with them and that they did design to kill all their head warriors." Such rumors were confirmed by other Natives and by the actions of traders who had been very abusive "and not as white men used to be to them."[118] Their own grievances thus made the Cherokees receptive to the message of revolt that the Yamasees carried to them just prior to the outbreak of the war.

The Cherokees' commitment to the revolt was weak at best, however. Soon after the conflict began, the English sent peace overtures, hoping to pry the largest of its former Native allies from the rebellion. Such an effort worked. Cherokees ceased their attacks by July and for doing so received a gift of over five hundred guns along with powder and shot.[119] The Cherokees warmly received the presents and sent a delegation to Charles Town in October to renew their kinship ties with the colony.[120] Carolinians hoped also to bring the Creeks back into a peaceful relationship and thus keep the French from taking over England's lucrative trading network that had reached all the way to the Mississippi. In December, Col. George Chicken with a force of three hundred men arrived at the Lower Cherokee town of Tugaloo with Carolina's plans for restoring peace.[121] Chicken found Cherokees divided. Lower Cherokees inclined for peace with the Creeks, while the other divisions of the nation seemed puzzled. Long-standing enmity between the two peoples existed and the English had enflamed the hostility by instigating Creek slave raids against Cherokees in 1706. The legacy of the Native slave trade would not go away easily. With peace, a spokesman for the Middle and Overhill Cherokees bluntly informed the English, "they should have no way in getting of slaves to buy ammunition & clothing."[122] A mysterious event ultimately determined the issue. Assailants murdered eleven Creek diplomats as they slept in the Tugaloo council house. The English claimed that Cherokees did this on their own initiative, but one Creek emissary was given to a Carolinian who promptly shot him, suggesting that Chicken's forces played some role in instigating the sordid affair.[123] In any event, the murders precipitated a conflict between the two indigenous nations that lasted nearly continuously for over forty years.

For their part, the English saw advantages in the Cherokee and Creek breach. They could not afford to completely side with the Cherokees, for if they did, French Louisiana's influence among the Creeks would grow. South Carolinians resorted to the strategy that served colonizers so well in the conquest of the Americas. They played one indigenous group off another. In June 1717, Carolinians received the delightful news that the Creeks were ready for peace with the English and resumption of trade. Carolinians immediately carried presents to the Lower Creeks, and then during the following fall Creek leaders traveled to Charles Town to conclude reconciliation. Early in 1718, Carolinian traders were once again traveling to the various Creek towns. Meanwhile, the Cherokees and Creeks remained at war. One Carolinian was quite candid in how such conflict benefited his colony. "To hold both as our friends, for some time, and assist them in cutting one another's throat without offending either," Joseph Boone revealed. "This is the game we intend to play . . . for if [we] cannot destroy one nation of Indians by another—our country must be lost."[124] Carolinians, to be sure, did not envision the Cherokee-Creek conflict as a means to perpetuate the Native slave trade; that noxious commerce resulted in the destructive Yamasee War and the few English traders who survived proved no longer willing to risk their lives and treasure on such an enterprise. Instead, they turned their attention almost exclusively to deerskins. The lesson of divide and conquer, however, had not been lost on Carolinians, and they used it successfully to keep their two most powerful allies from uniting.

The end of the Yamasee War left the Cherokees in a relationship with a duplicitous colony that supplied their enemies, but did it bring a round of smallpox? *Variola* certainly circulated in Charles Town in the spring and summer of 1718.[125] South Carolina's Commissioners of the Indian Trade worried that the disease would undermine the trading relations with their regained indigenous partners and ordered that Natives be warned to not come into Charles Town.[126] At the same time, though, they did not cut off traffic to their Native clients, particularly to their most powerful allies, the Cherokees. In mid-June the commissioners employed a trader and his five assistants to lead thirteen packhorses loaded with goods into southern Appalachia. After receiving reports that two hundred Frenchmen and many of their allied warriors had set out to attack the Cherokees, the commissioners authorized an additional supply of ammunition and a gunsmith to be sent to Tugaloo. They also sent advice "to in-fort their women and children" and alert the English if any Frenchmen came along with the suspected attack.[127] With a communication network linking southern Appalachia with smallpox-ridden Charles Town, with trade goods flowing to all divisions of their nation, and with their settlements being compactly organized for defense, conditions for an epidemic existed.

An outbreak, however, almost certainly did not happen. William Hatton, South Carolina's lead agent, resided among the Cherokees from 1717 to 1720 and soon thereafter wrote a narrative of his experience. He did not record anything suggestive of smallpox or an epidemic. It was likely the case then that the one condition absolutely necessary for an epidemic to occur was absent: a sizeable pool of individuals without acquired immunity. The Cherokees' previous exposure in 1698 and then possibly again in 1711 had left immunized survivors. What Cherokees in fact suffered most from during Hatton's stay was intertribal warfare that the colony of South Carolina enflamed. Late in 1718 or early 1719, one Creek attack resulted in the entire destruction of a Lower Cherokee town. The Creeks, according to Hatton, carried off an "abundance" of captives and "killed most of the rest of the inhabitants." Hatton further added that such attacks engendered much resentment toward the English. He relayed Cherokee views that "it was upon our accounts that they made war with the Creek Indians, depending on the promise of the white people to supply them plentifully with what they wanted but especially ammunition." Yet, the English not only failed to keep up their end of the bargain but also "made friends with the Creeks and stand fast by them," even giving them "a greater supply" of ammunition.[128] South Carolina, though, would continue to play the two indigenous nations against each other for decades to come, producing a harsh reality for its Native allies and making it difficult for both to sustain their populations amid colonialism's multiple traumas.

• • • •

By 1721, then, the Cherokees' population of 10,379 most likely did represent a fraction of what it had been before they developed sustained relations with the English, and a smallpox epidemic that occurred around 1698 probably played a major role in reducing them. But how big was that original—presmallpox—population? No census of the Cherokees exists documenting their numbers before the 1690s, thus making an answer to this question exceedingly difficult, if not impossible, to calculate.

One could attempt to derive pre-epidemic numbers by working backward from the known numbers that the British provided. One could choose a percentage of depopulation, subtract that from one hundred, and multiply the result by the 1721 total. But, the depopulation rate one chooses would inevitably be arbitrary since it would have to be based on a set of unknowable variables. First, one would have to know the mortality rate of smallpox. Epidemiologists cite that *Variola* took 40 percent of its victims in modern times, but one cannot know whether that accurately reflected what happened for indigenous populations living during the colonial era. "Virgin soil" theorists bandy about rates as high as 90 percent, but these seem incredibly high and based on the hyperbolic descriptions of colonial observers. Second, one would have to know how many Cherokees actually became infected. Widespread infection can be assumed based on the lack of acquired immunity and the general state of warfare that kept Native communities in a defensive posture during the height of the Native slave trade, but certainly some Cherokees escaped infection. Some were undoubtedly away from their villages hunting, gathering, or on diplomatic missions. Third, one would have to determine the net effect of captive raids. On one hand, Cherokees had multiple enemies that took people from their villages, but on the other hand they had considerable military strength and took many prisoners and adopted them. Assimilated Tuscaroras certainly made up some of the Cherokee population as did French inhabitants and

their Native allies from the Midwest. In 1715, for example, Cherokees took "a large number" of captives, including ten to twelve French
residents from the Illinois village of Kaskaskia, and attacked the
Cahokias, killing fifty warriors and sixteen French men and taking
all of their women and children as prisoners.[129] Whether Cherokees
conducted these raids as a conscious effort to augment their disease-
depleted communities is not known, but such activities would have
had that practical effect and thus masked depopulation due to disease.
Lastly, one would have to account for net reproduction rate. Cherokees certainly continued to have babies, but what was their normal
birth rate? Did they consciously try to increase rates due to losses
from disease? Or, did the traumas of colonialism interfere with fertility
and lead to further depression of their numbers? There is simply no
way to answer these multiple questions.

To derive a pre-epidemic population then one would have to
make several assumptions. Let us assume, for example, a simple case
scenario of a 40 percent mortality rate from smallpox, nearly universal infection, and no net population gain or loss through captive
raids or fluctuations of birth rates. In this case, the Cherokees had a
presmallpox population of 17,298. This number, though, appears
somewhat smaller than what other scholars have suggested. Anthropologist James Mooney proposed a population of 22,000 Cherokees
in the earliest study of Cherokee demography, while historian Peter
Wood more recently corrected these numbers upwards to a range of
30,000 to 35,000.[130] Both scholars make reasonable attempts, and their
respective estimates could be derived by manipulating the values
of the variables that affected population dynamics. In the end, one
must accept the uncertainty of pre-epidemic Cherokee numbers.
There could have been 17,000 or even fewer, or there could have
been as many as 32,500 or even more.[131]

Accepting this uncertainty allows our analysis of aboriginal depopulation to move into more fruitful directions: identifying the timing
of smallpox's arrival and reconstructing the larger historical context
in which it came. Great doubt exists regarding *Variola*'s hypothetical
spread throughout the Americas immediately following its 1518 introduction to Spain's Caribbean colonies. Cherokees especially did not
have extensive or intensive linkages with the world outside of their

southern Appalachian homeland until English colonialism dramatically transformed the Southeast. Until then, Cherokees were insulated from epidemics occurring even closer to them in New York or in Florida, and their own episodic encounters with Europeans—namely Hernando de Soto's and Juan Pardo's expeditionary forces—could not have introduced smallpox directly to them. At most, explorers helped plant malaria in a patchwork configuration in and around southern Appalachia, but virtually no chance existed that smallpox accompanied these interlopers. The likelihood of *Variola* reaching southern Appalachia increased over the course of the last half of the seventeenth century. Then, English commerce in Native slaves created a substantial increase in the flow of human traffic, which facilitated the transmission of smallpox across a vast region and created an intensely violent world in which Native peoples lived in compact, defensive settlements wherein universal infection became even more probable. It is indeed hard to imagine that Cherokees escaped the Great Southeastern Smallpox Epidemic. It struck their near neighbors particularly hard and the Cherokees' own oral history offers a vague recollection of the traumatic event.

The 10,379 Cherokees the English counted in the 1720s thus appear to be survivors of a larger population that had been reduced. No metaphors or figurative language, however, can adequately represent the causes of this reduction. To be sure, they at one time universally lacked acquired immunity but their vulnerability cannot be blamed entirely on their bodies. Their exposure to smallpox stemmed from English desires for Native slaves, desires that created a network that encompassed the southeastern region and its people and facilitated the spread of an acute infection. Following the Great Southeastern Smallpox Epidemic, colonialism did not abate: English commercial and imperial goals fueled the Tuscarora, Yamasee, and Creek Wars, which embroiled Cherokees in a cycle of violence that made population recovery difficult. Their population in the 1720s in other words reflected the consequences of living in a colonized world and not merely those of germs that supposedly spread like wildfire free of any human agency.

CHAPTER 2

RESPONSE

Becoming sick with a disease, sometimes severely so, was not something that happened only after Europeans arrived, and to deal with the frequent ailments and illnesses that bothered them, indigenous peoples did what human beings across the globe and throughout time have done: they practiced medicine. Medicine—the art of curing or preventing disease—is as an ancient activity and ubiquitous among human societies. Through the evolution of our species, people have performed acts to avoid illness and in the event of sickness have sought alleviation through the application of substances and other procedures aimed to restore health. The Cherokees of course were no exception. They had a rich medical tradition that developed well before Europeans ever arrived and had among them specially trained practitioners who diagnosed illnesses, attempted cures, and conducted rites to promote community health. Colonists most often referred to these individuals pejoratively as "conjurors" and sometimes more appropriately as "priests." But whatever they were called, Cherokees held them in high regard due to their important role in protecting people from harm.

But how did these individuals respond to smallpox? Ineptly, if one looks for an answer within the current body of historical works. Crosby claims that indigenous practitioners did not deal with contagious diseases and rejected the idea of quarantine until experiencing successive epidemics. In the meantime, their counterproductive actions "often had as decisive an influence on the death rate as did the virulency of the disease."[1] Other advocates of the "virgin soil"

thesis paint a dire picture as well, one in which indigenous medicine disintegrates in the wake of biological forces that Natives could
neither control nor understand. The historian William McNeill, for
example, claims that "stunned acquiescence in Spanish superiority
was the only possible response" for indigenous peoples in the wake
of epidemics in Latin America. He adds that "Native authority
structures crumbled; the old gods seemed to have abdicated. . . .
Docility to the commands of priests, viceroys, . . . and anyone else
who spoke with a loud voice and had a white skin was another inevitable consequence."[2] Axtell also suggests declension and acculturation.
He characterizes indigenous shamans as "totally impotent" in the
wake of epidemics that swept Canada during French colonization.
Jesuit missionaries subsequently "rushed forward with free nursing,
comforting if not curative medicines, and plausible theological explanation for the misfortunes that had taken the natives unawares."[3]
Other scholars make the same conclusions that Native healers responded
ineffectively, their leadership became questioned, and Europeans
consequently implanted their culture.[4]

The anthropologist Calvin Martin proposes the most novel interpretation of Native response to epidemics, but one that also characterizes practitioners as impotent in the wake of colonialism's biological
consequences. He begins with the question of why Natives of eastern
Canada participated in the fur trade, an enterprise that led them to
overhunt game animals that they relied upon for food and clothing.
Hunters did this, Martin concludes, not simply to exchange their pelts
and hides to Europeans for material goods but to exact revenge on
the beings thought responsible for terrible epidemics. Indigenous
peoples commonly believed spiritual guardians of animals could
afflict humans with disease when taboos such as overhunting were
violated, but the epidemics exceeded any proper retaliation against
hunters for such transgressions. Humans were thus freed to wage a
war of extermination. Epidemics, moreover, rendered shamans "powerless to mend the shattered universe" and restore traditional taboos.
Ordinary people saw their shaman's "ability to control and otherwise
influence the supernatural realm dysfunctional—because his magic
and other traditional cures were now ineffective."[5] In the end, epidemics had "triggered the secularization or profanation of the aboriginal

spiritual world" and opened the door for the acculturative aspects of colonialism, namely trade dependency and Christianity.[6]

The belief that Native practitioners responded ineptly and that epidemics led to cultural declension has also made its way into Cherokee historiography. To be sure, no one has argued, and it would be absurd to do so, that Cherokee medicine disappeared. It has obviously survived—practitioners retained traditional knowledge, conducted various rites and ceremonies, and continued to work with patients well into the nineteenth century, and they still do so today in some communities in Oklahoma and North Carolina. Such survival has led to a particularly rich body of ethnographic information that missionaries and professional anthropologists have collected. Nevertheless, William McLoughlin—one of the most prolific scholars of Cherokee history—has given novel germs some credit for disorienting Cherokees from their traditional customs and beliefs. "The remedies tried by their medicine men often simply hastened the death of the victims," McLoughlin wrote in reference to James Adair's depiction of the 1738–39 epidemic. "This failure of their doctors/priests tended to erode faith in them and their rituals. . . . Tribal animosity against the priests resulted in what seems to have been a repudiation of them and their methods, perhaps even their assassination." He then refers his readers to "a former priestly hierarchy" that Cherokees believed "existed in olden times" but had disappeared by the early nineteenth century.[7] His work thus follows in line with the "virgin soil" thesis in that Native personnel at best preserved their medicine when it came to aboriginal illnesses but proved to be counterproductive or fatalistic when it came to introduced diseases and consequently suffered a loss of status. McLoughlin claims, as a matter of fact and without citing any source, that "the services of their medicine men were not considered effective against whitemen's diseases like measles and smallpox."[8]

McLoughlin's conclusions in particular as well as those within the historical literature in general, however, have not been subject to much scholarly scrutiny. Such scrutiny is long overdue. Regarding the Cherokees' experience with smallpox, a critical and in-depth look at James Adair's passage on the 1738–39 epidemic reveals the limitations in using widely cited anecdotes and privileging them without careful analysis and without considering other evidence. A more complete picture can be discerned by putting Cherokee responses into the context of the early modern world of medicine, one before knowledge of viruses and bacteria existed, vaccines to prevent primary infections had been developed, and antibiotics to fight secondary infections had been invented. In such a world, the best medicine anyone—European or Native—could practice was to avoid communities where the disease circulated, and, if exposure did occur, offer simple nursing care to the infected, enact quarantine to prevent the spread of contagion, and promote calmness and solidarity so that basic social services such as gathering food, water, and firewood did not break down. A wider array of evidence in other words can be brought to bear to demonstrate that there is much more to be known about Native responses to colonialism's most dreaded germ than what the "virgin soil" thesis's sweeping generalizations misleadingly teach.

• • • •

Cherokees drew upon an elaborate system of preexisting beliefs and practices about medicine when they confronted smallpox. Unfortunately a scholar can only know about this system through imperfect information. Eighteenth-century colonial observers captured only glimpses of medical practices and left only scattered bits of detail about it. Information is more voluminous through the records of the Protestant missionary Daniel Butrick, who left posterity with several volumes of ethnographic information he acquired in the 1820s and 1830s from informants that had recently converted or who considered doing so.[9] Such information, however, was often filtered through a Judeo-Christian lens, which distorted Cherokee beliefs in multiple spirit beings to fit a monotheistic world view. Richer and more nuanced information comes in the late nineteenth century with the work of the professional anthropologist James Mooney. As did his professional peers at the time, Mooney sought to make a permanent record of Native beliefs and customs, which he thought existed in an unchanged form from the time before Europeans arrived. Such information also has its drawbacks. Native peoples certainly lost knowledge and abandoned practices as well as accepted new ideas and customs from outside groups. Mooney at times failed to distinguish between original and introduced cultural forms. Nevertheless, such imperfect information—whether it came from an off-handed comment by an eighteenth-century colonist, a letter by an ethnocentric missionary, or a naive anthropologist—does not preclude any understanding of what Cherokees believed and practiced before they developed sustained relations with Europeans. Taken altogether and critically read, the information can offer a plausible cultural baseline from which to proceed to the larger analysis on how Cherokees responded to smallpox.[10]

Hereditary descent figures prominently in the information available on Cherokee medicine. Ordinary people may have acquired some medical skill over the course of their lifetimes, but the most esteemed practitioners came from particular lineages that possessed a special repository of knowledge. A Cherokee priest, for example, explained to the English trader Alexander Longe in the 1710s that a certain physic family supplied practitioners for his community. The priest told Longe that he belonged to this family and as a young boy became an apprentice to an elder, who trained him in information that had been passed "from generation to generation by their ancestors." Longe's informant added that he himself had selected some of his young relatives and taught "them all sort of doctoring" and examined them "every new moon."[11] The pupils learned prayers, songs, and formulas that they used to mediate with the spirit world and conducted this mediation with what Longe called "a lingo or gibberish" that none could understand but those trained in its use.[12]

More details about the inherited nature of medicine can be found in Butrick's records. Some children, the missionary learned, had "hereditary rights" to practice medicine and began an apprenticeship at an early age. Under the guidance of an elder, each apprentice underwent intense training involving seclusion in the woods, fasting, and purification and along the way acquired an awareness of the various spiritual beings that existed throughout the cosmos, how to call upon them in times of need, how to read signs and omens, and how to lead followers in various rites. Practitioners carefully guarded what they had learned, believing its efficacy would be diminished if revealed to individuals unprepared for it. Of particular importance was the care and use of a special quartz-stone implement, known as an "ulv-sata." Practitioners used this object to perform divination in certain ceremonial contexts, and they entrusted it to no one except their most qualified apprentices who would inherit it upon their deaths.[13]

That family connections were important for one to become a medical practitioner did not mean that a single lineage ever monopolized religious activities among Cherokees. Several lineages certainly had medical knowledge and skill, and most likely these families existed within each of the Cherokees' seven clans. If members of one particular community became dissatisfied with practitioners that lived among them, moreover, they sought more suitable individuals from other lineages and even from other communities. In addition, medical practitioners had to share the stage with other religious leaders who conducted various rites that Cherokees saw as necessary for survival. Mediation with the spirit world was also seen as necessary for warfare, horticulture, and hunting, and while some individuals may have practiced in multiple realms, specialization occurred. Some practitioners utilized their knowledge and skills to mediate with the spirit world in just the rites of warfare, for example. Priests skilled in treating and preventing diseases in other words did not constitute the only spiritual leadership for their people.[14]

Medical practitioners also existed within a decentralized political structure in which power was dispersed among more secular leaders as well. Some warriors achieved high status and earned the title of Raven. These served as the war chief of their town or at times multiple towns and often took a leading role in negotiating with Europeans. Another high-status individual was referred to as "Uka." Alexander Longe called these individuals "kings" in the earliest account of Cherokee political structure and described them as being separate from "priests." Kings were served first during communal feasts but did not perform the rites involved in such events. Several other English observers directly identified Ukas as secular town leaders. The English trader Ludovick Grant, who started living among the Cherokees in 1726 and narrated his experience in 1756, characterized an Uka as essentially a first among equals rather than a monarch that ruled by divine right.[15] The Scottish visitor Alexander Cuming learned in 1730 that Ukas were "elected out of certain families," implying some hereditary leadership among the Cherokees, but the Scot commented that this head leader was "little else than a Civil Magistrate." No evidence furthermore indicates that a single Uka ever led the entire Cherokees Nation, although some powerful civil leaders emerged who had influence that encompassed multiple towns. Cuming also noted that at times the Uka could be a great warrior, demonstrating that the Cherokees did not divide power as rigidly between civil and military leaders as did some other indigenous groups.[16] A war chief in other words could become an Uka, a fact evidenced by the leadership during the American Revolution of Savanukeh, a man whom English speakers called "the Raven of Chota."[17]

Butrick's records flesh out the decentralized leadership structure among Cherokees. The missionary found no evidence of an Uka playing a leading role in mediating with the spirit world. Instead, the Uka gave his consent to when certain ceremonies would be performed but did not conduct the rites involved. The role of these headmen then seemed to be a spokesperson for his community, one who gathered the advice from a variety of individuals including practitioners and who articulated a consensus view of his people.[18] Much of this advice came from a town council of representatives from each of the seven clans. Known as Beloved Men, these individuals achieved high regard through their service to the community and then served as mediators between the more secular authority of the Uka and more sacred authority of practitioners.[19] Beloved Men also resided near the council house, kept track of the cycles of the moon, decided when the people were to plant, determined when certain ceremonies would take place, and assisted practitioners in ceremonial preparations. At times, Beloved Men even selected which practitioners would preside over specific ceremonies.[20]

A medical practitioner thus was one among many leaders in the decentralized and relatively egalitarian Cherokee Nation. Still, they commanded respect, exercised influence over a range of issues that their communities faced, and in doing so drew the attention of Europeans. "Their conjurers are the persons consulted in every affair of importance, and seem to have the direction of everything," Cuming recorded.[21] Similarly, a Christian minister, who made a brief visit during the winter of 1758–59, found Cherokees largely uninterested in the Gospel, lamenting, "They are much given to conjuring & the conjurers have great power over [them]."[22] A British army officer also had his plans frustrated due to a practitioner's influence. In 1756, he armed the Overhill leader Attakullakulla and his men for an attack against the French, but they returned home early without reaching their target. "They intended to have continued out three months," the officer learned, "but their conjurors' prognosticating that they should lose some of the warriors as well as kill some of the Enemy they thought it the best to return and preserve their lives of their people."[23] Two years later, Attakullakulla again frustrated his allies with his deference to his spiritual advisors who told him to stay home rather than go out against Great Britain's enemies. The Cherokee man explained that "they never undertook anything of consequence, but they consulted their conjurers to know the pleasure of the Great Man above and they never departed from his opinion."[24]

These powerful practitioners were not necessarily always male, although Europeans almost always identified them as such. In general, females had more power in Cherokee society than they did in neighboring English settlements. Women did things that English women would not have dared to do. Female Cherokees sat in councils, publically expressed their views on important matters such as war and peace, determined the fate of captives, and took part in diplomatic missions. To be sure, a division of labor existed between males and females within Cherokee society. Horticulture—planting, tending, and harvesting the crops—was the domain of women, while hunting and warfare remained the domain of men.[25] The division of the sexes in medicine, though, was a bit more complicated. Young girls certainly learned esoteric knowledge from their elders and as they grew older became active practitioners. Patriarchal Europeans often failed to notice such females. The British officer Alexander Cameron, however, proved to be an exception. He labeled the female leader of Keowee as "the greatest conjuror" in the Cherokee Nation at the time of her death in 1773.[26] It is not certain whether this individual presided over medical, horticultural, war ceremonies, or all. In any event, other sources suggest distinct roles that male and female practitioners played in Cherokee rituals. Each town had a council of seven Beloved Women,

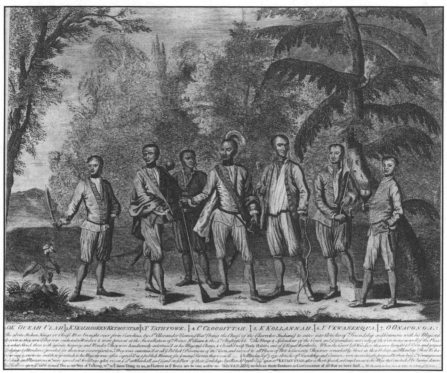

The Chiefs of the Cherokee Indians, copperplate engraving by Isaac Basire (ca. 1730). As a young man, Attakullakulla (far right) joined six other Cherokee leaders on a visit to London where they met with King George II. Attakullakulla strove to keep his people allied to the British throughout his life, but he still followed the guidance of Cherokee practitioners when considering options for his people during the colonial era. (Courtesy of the Collection of the Museum of Early Southern Decorative Arts, Old Salem Museums and Gardens)

representatives from each clan who had gained the high esteem of their kinsmen. As with their male counterparts, the Beloved Women advised the Uka about the proper time to convene communal rituals, made preparations for particularly important ceremonies, and fulfilled key functions in these.[27]

• • • •

Whether male or female, a practitioner approached medicine with a complex understanding of the cosmos and the powers that infused it. While the particular details about these powers may have varied from practitioner to practitioner and changed over time, the rich ethnographic sources from the colonial period through the nineteenth century demonstrate deep cultural persistence regarding cosmology, one in which Cherokees conceived of themselves as inhabiting a terrestrial world filled with both visible creatures and invisible spirits. This world, moreover, existed in between an upper and a lower world, each of which served as the dwelling place of numerous beings that affected the day-to-day lives of humans and animals. No spirit or being in any of the three levels was inherently good or evil, but altogether they were a quarrelsome lot. They existed in tension with each other and often acted antagonistically toward one another. They kept the cosmos in a continual state of flux and produced much danger that kept people constantly on their guard.[28]

The most powerful spirits with which Cherokees dealt resided in the upper world. The sun, moon, thunders, and winds, for example, were each conceived of as beings with creative and destructive powers. They brought forth the produce of the earth through rain and sunshine but could withhold the rains or bring deadly storms and torrential downpours. The ancestral spirits of the animals also existed in the upper world. Humans killed the progeny of these spirits for food and clothing and in doing so risked offending their guardians in the upper world. The corn mother, Selu, also resided in the upper world. She ascended to the eastern sky after providing maize for people and showing them how to cultivate this life-sustaining crop. Her husband, Kana'ti, came to live with her after teaching his hunting techniques to his two mischievous sons, who then disobeyed him and let loose the game that he kept enclosed in a cave. The rebellious sons thereafter lived in the western sky as thunder beings known as the Little Men. Such beliefs encouraged Cherokees themselves to be obedient to Kana'ti's and Selu's lessons and to call upon them for aid.[29]

The lower world also had its share of spirits. Cherokees believed that rivers originated in a powerful underworld, one of fertility and healing but also mystery and danger. Springs that fed rivers were thought to be portals into this world through which spirits could pass back and forth. A river itself was conceived of as a being called Long Man, who provided humans with purifying and healing powers

and deserved respect and devotion.[30] More dangerous to the Cherokees was another being of the lower world, the Uktena. The thunders
of the upper world created the ancestor of these serpent-like creatures to destroy the sun. Having failed, the Uktena descended to earth
and left its spawn in "deep pools in the river and about lonely passes
in the high mountains."[31] Each of these creatures had horns on its
head, a single crystal for an eye, the body of a snake with bright red
scales, and wings. Ordinary humans greatly feared encountering one
of these creatures, but the Cherokees maintained a tradition that
powerful medical practitioners occasionally confronted an Uktena,
acquired its crystal eye, and made it his ulvsata.[32]

Cherokees lived in tension with spirits in the terrestrial world as
well. They believed their deceased kinsmen existed in spiritual form
but wanted to hold onto their place among the living. Before making
their departure to their destination in the western sky—the Darkening Land—they often dwelt near where they had lived, seeking to
take their loved ones with them.[33] Even from the Darkening Land,
lonely spirits sought out the companionship of their kinsmen by
visiting them in their dreams. Other spiritual beings, which might
take the form of humans but who were not fully human, were believed
to exist in the world that humans inhabited. The Nanehi, for example, split their time between the lower world and the surface world.
During the day they lived in the water, ground, and mountains but
came out at night and then could be seen. Cherokees described some
of these as being small in "the shape of people" but having "eyes
projected, as if on the ends of horns" and others as bigger with long
eyes "extending up & down." In general, the Nanehi were helpful
but could be vengeful if not shown proper respect.[34]

Disrespected beings indeed proved dangerous. Mooney's informants told him, "In the old days, quadrupeds, birds, fishes and insects
could all talk, and they and the human race lived together in peace
and friendship." But the people began to grow more numerous and
invented "bows, knives, blowguns, spears, and hooks" to kill the large
animals, while "the smaller creatures, such as the frogs and worms,
were crushed and trodden upon without mercy." The deer took action
to stop such mistreatment and under the leadership of their "chief"
Little Deer they decided to "inflict rheumatism upon every hunter

who should kill one of their number, unless he took care to ask their pardon for the offense." From that point on, Little Deer always went to the spot in which a deer was killed and asked the spirit of the slain creature if the hunter had prayed for a pardon. If not, then the guardian followed the hunter to his home and inflicted him with a crippling disease that ruined his ability to hunt again.[35] Similarly, the ancestors to snakes and fishes grew upset at human depredations and "determined to make their victims dream of snakes twining about them in slimy folds and blowing their fetid breath in their faces, or to make them dream of eating raw or decaying fish, so that they would lose appetite, sicken, and die."[36] Small insects and worms also took exception to being "crushed, burned or otherwise destroyed through the unthinking carelessness of the human race." The ghosts of these animals took vengeance and established towns "under the skin of their victims, thus producing an irritation which results in fevers, boils, scrofula and other diseases."[37]

The guardians of animals were not the only beings thought to inflict disease upon people. Spirits of the upper world could sicken people below them. Butrick, although condensing Cherokee conceptions of the upper world into a monotheistic frame, learned from his informants that "when God was displeased with any people, He sent sickness by means of . . . the fire, the water, the moon, or the thunder."[38] In another story the missionary recorded that Selu could use disease to chastise humans. The corn mother warned her children to carefully tend the gift she gave them and pay her proper respect: "But if you forget to think of me and these things . . . [and] if you should take no heed, but make use of me without remembering my words, I will fling among you . . . disease, distress, anguish, the destroyer."[39]

A more elaborate story puts disease into the context of a drama involving the sun, the moon, the thunders, and the Uktena. Mooney recorded, "Now, the Sun hated the people on the earth because they could never look straight at her without screwing up their faces." Her brother, the moon, however, looked fondly upon humans for they "always smiled pleasantly" at him. The sun's jealousy led her to take drastic action. Everyday around noon, she caused a great fever through her burning rays that killed a great many. The Little Men decided to help the suffering people and transformed two men into snakes—the spreading adder and the copperhead—to bite the sun when she stopped to visit her daughter. These creatures failed in the mission, leading the Little Men to transform a man into a more dangerous being, the Uktena. But this creature too failed to stop the sun, leading the two thunders to create the rattlesnake to do the job. Jealous of this new creature, the Uktena "grew angrier all the time and very dangerous, so that if he even looked at a man, that man's family would die."[40] The rattlesnake managed to get the sun to cease killing the people, but not exactly as the Little Men had planned. The rattlesnake accidently bit and killed the sun's daughter. While in mourning, the sun ceased sending her sickening rays onto the people and all became dark. The people worried they would never see the sun return and again appealed to the Little Men for help. The two thunders told the humans they must retrieve the sun's daughter from the Darkening Land, put her in a box, and bring her back to her mother without opening the box. The humans succeeded in capturing the spirit of the girl but succumbed to her pleas to be let out. She immediately escaped in the form of a redbird. The Little Men admonished the people, telling them that since they did not bring the sun's daughter home safely, they would never be able to retrieve anyone once they died. The deceased, in other words, would forever reside in the Darkening Land.[41]

Not only did humans have to accept mortality as a consequence of their actions but they also had to continue to deal with the Little Men's creations—snakes and the Uktena. Rattlesnakes in particular retained a connection to the thunders.[42] Cherokees referred to such a creature as "the thunder's necklace" and believed that "to kill one is to destroy one of the most prized ornaments of the thunder god." Rattlesnakes, nonetheless, were generally thought to be "kind" beings who could be prayed to for aid and who would not harm unless humans disturbed them.[43] The Uktena was more dangerous. After failing to kill the sun, the creature left his progeny on earth, and these hid in the lower world.[44] If anyone encountered an Uktena, "certain death" would result.[45] Their blood and scales were thought to be so poisonous that contact with either would instantly kill a person. Capturing the Uktena's crystal on its forehead could bring an individual great power but mishandling it could result in serious harm. Cherokee practitioners who possessed one of these objects protected them from the touch of ordinary people and fed it with the blood of small game every seven days and the blood of a deer or other large animal twice a year. Failure to maintain such care would lead an Uktena to take vengeance. The Cherokees believed that "it would come out from its cave at night in a shape of fire and fly through the air to slake its thirst with the lifeblood of the conjurer or some one of his people."[46]

While mythic beings of ancient origin such as the Uktena figure prominently in Cherokee stories about disease, human beings themselves, both the living and the dead, could act as agents of sickness, suffering, and even death. The spirits of the deceased, for example, longed for the companionship of their kinsmen and visited them through dreams in an effort to lure them to the afterlife.[47] They did so not out of malevolence but rather loneliness. Cherokees consequently avoided discussion of the dead, lest one encouraged deceased relatives into his or her dreams. In the event that a dream involving a dead person occurred, the dreamer would seek out the counsel of a medical practitioner even before symptoms appeared.[48]

A more malevolent means of inducing sickness involved living humans who chose to use their medicine to harm others. Beliefs in what we might call wizardry or witchcraft were widespread among indigenous peoples, and references to such beliefs can be found in colonial era documents as well as in later ethnographic materials. Witches, according to the Cherokees, did not serve as the original cause of disease but rather practiced bad medicine to turn the spirit world against other people. These witches, moreover, could act clandestinely. They turned themselves into animals, especially birds, so that their malevolent actions would escape detection. Often these beings came upon victims who were already suffering from disease and stole their life from them, thus adding years onto their own existence and allowing them to live to be quite old.[49]

• • • •

With a diverse array of beings potentially involved in causing disease, Cherokee practitioners approached healing by first attempting to discern clues from the spirit world. Their patient's symptoms provided little help in making diagnoses and in fact might have been misleading, since beings attempted to trick practitioners by inflicting a different set of ailments in different circumstances.[50] One spirit might, for example, cause dysentery in one individual and ulcerated skin in another, while two different spirits might cause the same symptoms in two separate individuals. Medicine thus was not a matter of matching symptoms to a fixed and known culprit but a process of discovering evidence left by any one of a number of fickle beings and then appealing to other spirits for aid.[51]

Dreams and omens provided the best clues for practitioners to diagnosis a disease. Cherokee ethnography is filled with examples of what practitioners might have learned from their interviews with their patients. If a patient informed his doctor that he dreamed of seeing snakes, for example, the physician might conclude that "it is a sign that that snake, by witchcraft, has occasioned the sickness."[52] Other dreams portended sickness. An ill patient or an individual who expects to become sick might reveal for example that he or she dreamed of a rising stream, a dead animal, water rising around a house, or their clothes being on fire.[53] Some dreams foretold death for the dreamer or a family member, including those in which the dreamer sees himself or someone else walking toward the west, going down a stream of high water, or holding an eagle's feather. If the dreamer saw a house burning or an eagle on the ground, then someone was surely going to die soon. The practitioner also listened closely to discover whether his patient or a family member encountered any anomalous behaviors of animals. If a family member revealed that he began a journey and observed a fox take a few steps, stop, look back, and bark, the practitioner might conclude "that some one of his family, or neighbors would die before his return or soon after." Other omens included a whip-poor-will coming near a house and repeatedly singing; two squirrels fighting and one consequently falling from a tree; a dog talking like a person; a screech owl making "some uncommon noise"; and a tree falling without wind.[54]

Dreams and omens served as windows into the spirit world, but they might not have revealed enough information. Practitioners had to use their own communicative abilities. To discover whether their medicine might be effective, they might apply an animal's blood to their divining crystals and look for particular images to appear. Or, they might sacrifice a deer's tongue to the fire and listen to the way in which the meat popped and observe the direction and color of the smoke that was produced. Practitioners could also use examining beads. They would put different colored beads in their hands and move the beads between their fingers. Through such means, practitioners hoped to gain important information about the spirits that had made their patients sick, including their symbolic colors, locations, and possible collaborators.[55]

After determining the identity of the likely culprit, the healer sought the aid of spirits that would be particularly useful against those of the disease-causing agent. In general this aid came from beings whose powers countervailed those of the spirit that caused the disorder. If worms were suspected, for example, then the physician might begin with a prayer to the birds for a cure.[56] Or, if the west wind was suspected, then the physician prayed to the east wind and utilized plants whose roots grew in an easterly direction.[57] Other cures called for an appeal to the spirits that had a mythic connection to what caused the disease. If snakes were involved, for example, then a practitioner might appeal to the Little Men to take the snakes for themselves since they adorned themselves with these creatures.[58] In other instances, the practitioner gathered substances that had anomalous yet powerful characteristics. Bark from a tree that had been broken but continued to grow might be useful against crippling diseases. Similarly, lightning-struck wood would bring special curative powers, especially if the tree withstood its injury and continued to survive.[59] Bark from evergreen trees, ginseng roots, and other materials that came from plant life that did not seem to die during the winter were especially thought to have a connection with powerful spirits. These spirits, rather than the substances in themselves, were thought to be the curative agents.[60]

Whichever materials practitioners chose, they relied on mediums of water and fire to give their treatment potency.[61] Recall that streams served as a connector to the lower world, a mystical place where multiple spirits dwelled. By steeping their medicines in spring waters that fed streams, practitioners tapped the powers of the lower world to enhance their medical decoctions. Practitioners, moreover, almost always included in their treatment a bathing rite called "Going-to-Water." This involved the practitioners leading their patients into a nearby river and having them plunge seven times alternately in the directions of east and west. In doing so, the priest called upon Long Man to use his purifying powers to take diseases away and distribute them elsewhere.

Fire on the other hand connected humans to the upper world. The thunders had sent fire to the earth for the first time by way of lightning. Cherokees thereafter revered fire as an active agent of the thunders and believed its smoke served as means to transport their appeals to upper world spirits.[62] Hunters, for example, waived their moccasins and leggings over the fire for aid against poisonous snakes—creatures that had a special connection to the Little Men that created them and to whom the hunters' prayers were certainly addressed.[63] Similarly, medical practitioners offered sacrifices to the fire, usually a deer's tongue accompanied by tobacco sprinkles, to pay reverence to upper world spirits. They also boiled their medicines over the sacred flames and sent their appeals upward via smoke and steam to the particular beings they believed would empower their medicine.[64]

Throughout a treatment, healers strictly observed taboos, acted with reciprocity, and demanded their patients and family members do so as well. Practitioners prayed to the spirit of the materials they obtained and gave gifts. Where plants were taken from the ground, for example, they dropped beads in the cavity and covered them with soil.[65] Practitioners sought to further protect the strength of their medicine by having patients and their kinsmen distance themselves from anything associated with the spirit that caused the disease. Someone being treated for rheumatism, for example, did not consume rabbit meat because of the animal's hunchback appearance, while family members removed feathers from the home of a patient suffering from a disease that spirits of the birds caused.[66] Anyone thought to be unclean was also kept away from patients. Menstruating women, wounded warriors, and other individuals who could not control the emanation of their bodily fluids were especially forbidden from contact with patients. Ordinarily segregated from the larger community, such individuals could pollute the efficacy of a variety of rituals especially medical practices. More ominously, an individual who had contact with a dead person could undermine the physician's treatment and had to stay away from others until undergoing ritual purification.[67] If all went well and the patient recovered, a final act of reciprocity had to occur. The patient and his family were expected to give a gift to the physician. Failure to do so was an offense not only to the practitioner but also to the spiritual agents called upon to give efficacy to the treatment employed.[68]

In the event the healer was unsuccessful, a variety of outcomes might result. When their patients remained alive, practitioners might conclude that multiple agents worked together to produce the disease and would proceed to employ different medicines. Healers might also conclude that they lacked the required skill in curing an individual and would recommend another practitioner.[69] In the event that a physician lost a patient, he or she discontinued the practice of medicine until undergoing ritual purification at the time of the next new moon.[70] In some cases, the deceased patient's family might hold the practitioner responsible for the death and exact vengeance.[71] In such cases, physicians were believed to be malevolent witches or wizards rather than beneficent healers. The most skilled practitioners, however, avoided accusations of witchcraft, either by refusing to take patients that they believed had a good chance of dying or by deflecting blame onto others for employing bad medicine in opposition to their efforts to cure.

• • • •

Administering treatment to an individual patient, however, was only one aspect of a medical practitioner's role. Indigenous peoples saw their health and well-being as a collective affair, and they called upon individuals most knowledgeable about the spiritual world to lead them in various rites.[72] These aimed at establishing reciprocal relationships between people and the various beings of the cosmos, thereby protecting communities from chaos, disorder, and harm.

Cherokee life revolved around at least five major ceremonies, each associated with a pivotal moment in the seasonal cycle. As the grasses began to sprout in March and the planting season approached, people gathered in their communities to practice the First New Moon Festival.

Thereafter they prepared their fields, planted their crops, and guarded them against pests and scavengers. By late June or early July, they again convened and celebrated the Green Corn Ceremony, an event timed to the appearance of the first crop of edible maize. They observed another Green Corn Ceremony in August or early September when crops fully ripened and maize kernels began to harden. With the harvest completed and the leaves beginning to change colors, communities practiced the Great New Moon Festival, an event that marked the time in which the world was created and a time that Cherokees believed a new year commenced. Around a week later, they gathered again to celebrate the Atohvna, an event involving intense purification of both spaces and bodies.[73] A break in the calendar occurred during the late fall and winter as hunting consumed the attention of Cherokees. As the weather began to warm and signs of spring emerged, the ceremonial cycle began anew. At each of these key moments, Cherokees believed that the spirits must not be taken for granted and that respect must be shown to them through carefully planned and conducted rituals.

The Atohvna in particular had an association with health and medicine and deserves close attention. A town's Beloved Men appointed the time in which this ceremony would commence and gave its presiding priest the name "Unawisanvhi," which means "one who renews heart and body, or cleanses from mental and bodily defilements." The priest was also referred to as "Ulistuli," meaning "one who has his head covered," due to the special headdress he wore. Devoted since infancy to understanding the spirit world, the Ulistuli was looked upon as "a preacher of righteousness, teaching all moral duties." He possessed an ulvsata, which he carried with him in a necklace made of an animal skin bag.[74] The priest did not officiate alone, however. He had his apprentice or right-hand man by his side at all times and a singer, appointed by the Beloved Men and known as the "Yowatikanogisti." This latter individual was yet another individual trained from an early age in sacred knowledge and once appointed as a singer he retained his title of Yowatikanogisti for life.[75] Representatives from each of the seven clans, moreover, were appointed to perform special tasks in the week-long preparation for the event and throughout the four days of the ceremony itself.

The Atohvna involved a lengthy process of planning and execution. One week before the ceremony was to begin, the Beloved Men sent their town's most skilled hunters out to acquire meat for the gathering. Other community members were appointed to cleanse the council house and town dwellings, another group to gather the plant materials that would be ritually prepared for communal consumption, and a third group to tend to the fire to be used during the ceremony. Meanwhile, the lead practitioner and his assistants maintained a fast during the preparations, abstaining from food except only a light meal consumed daily after sunset. On the night before the Atohvna began, all community members arrived and the women commenced a special dance that lasted late into the evening. The first full day was devoted to intensive purification and divination as well as feasting and dancing during the night, although the priests and his assistants still only consumed a light meal after ordinary people ate. During the second and third days, the priest's assistants distributed venison from the communal stores, and the people ate as they pleased, again with the exception of the priest and his assistants maintaining their fast. The fourth day was much like the first, but all kept awake and women danced until the morning. At sunrise, the community members left the council house, one by one following the lead of the priest and his assistants and with this the Atohvna came to an end.

Throughout the Atohvna, strict purity was maintained. The clan representatives who tended the fire, for example, fed the flames with seven different types of wood, all of which came directly from trees rather than the ground where worms, insects, and other contaminants existed.[76] Women extinguished the fires in their homes, disposed of the ashes, and cleansed their fire places. Each then retrieved flame from the council house, started a new fire, and sacrificed a piece of meat. To keep unwelcomed spirits away, clan representatives whipped the eves of the council house and the town's other buildings with rods made from white sycamore trees. Such efforts aimed to chase away mischievous beings that might through jealousy undermine the town's efforts to build good relations with the spirit world. Throughout the preparation and performance of the ceremony, individuals who might inadvertently ruin their community's efforts were also kept away. Just as in cases of individual healing, people emitting bodily fluids and individuals who had recently come into close contact with the dead had to remain separate, although they could have some of the ceremonial food taken to them.

The key component of the Atohvna involved communal consumption of medicine. The priest's assistants placed a large pot over the new fire and filled it with spring water. The priest himself continued the ritual preparation by walking completely around the pot, sprinkling tobacco on the fire, and waving a white heron's wing, which dispersed the steamy smoke "in every direction," and praying. He did this four times to pay reverence to each wind that blew from the respective cardinal directions. The priest then ordered an assistant to place into the pot an array of bark, sprigs, and roots that had been carefully selected prior to the ceremony. Each of these plant materials had a close relationship with a spiritual power just as did materials that medical practitioners utilized when treating individuals. One Cherokee listed these items as those that do not die during the winter: cedar, white pine, hemlock, mistletoe, evergreen briar, heart leaf, and ginseng root. Another listed willow roots as an ingredient but only those that sprung from trees near a stream and stretched into the water.[77] Such roots almost certainly were believed to carry the power of Long Man.[78] After the contents came together and brewed for some time, clan leaders dipped their gourds into the concoction and delivered it to their respective kin groups. The people consumed the sacred beverage and washed their children's breast and their own with it as well. In this medicine, beings from all three levels of the cosmos united—spring water from the lower world, fire and smoke from the upper world, and plant life from the terrestrial world—thus bringing the Cherokees spiritual aid to live in a world filled with tensions and antagonisms.

Following consumption of this medicine, on the first day, the people underwent further purification with the Going-to-Water rite, a practice incorporated into other major ceremonies as well as a stand-alone practice between annual events. Before midmorning, the priest led the people to the river, prayed for them, and ordered them into the water. Each individual plunged entirely underwater seven times. They were not to wipe the water off their faces because the practice, meant to do more than simply rid the body of filth, cleansed the mind as well. The Long Man's powers were thought to "ward off the evil presaged by dreams of sudden death" and spells of "some secret enemy."[79] Some participants discarded their old clothes and allowed the stream to carry them away, while all changed into new clothes when coming out of the river and before returning to the council house. Such intensive ritual activity, which occurred again on the fourth day, led Cherokees to believe that after the Atohvna they had achieved their highest level of purity during the entire cycle of seasons.

Such purity was not a certain guard against misfortune, however. The priest alerted his followers to this reality by employing the art of divination. After returning from the river, the presiding priest sacrificed the tongue of the first buck killed in preparation for the Atohvna. He placed the tongue on the coals of the sacred fire and carefully watched and listened. Butrick records: "As many times as the meat popped, so many deaths would occur during the year. In case there was to be much sickness among the people, the smoke of the sacrifice would form a bluish cloud over the fire and not rise directly; otherwise it would arise directly towards heaven." The priest employed at least one other method of divining during the Atohvna. He placed his ulvsata on each of seven folded deerskins and prayed. If "a bright blaze without smoke appeared in the stone," then the community could expect a healthy year, but if the priest observed a "smoky appearance, . . . as many as were to die with the sickness would appear in the right side of it."[80] Such ominous predictions undoubtedly alerted people to the necessity of maintaining reciprocity with the spiritual powers that existed all around them.[81]

Cherokees thus had no illusions that the Atohvna would itself bring about an idyllic world of health, well-being, and harmony.[82] They lived in a universe ridden with antagonisms and tensions among competing spiritual powers that if not shown proper respect could harm humans. But the Atohvna and other major ceremonies would certainly ameliorate conflicts and enhance human fortunes. Practiced at key moments of change in their seasonal cycle, annual ceremonies then represented the best preventative medicine, or as Butrick recorded, Cherokees practiced the Atohvna so "that God might defend them from all sickness and unforeseen evils."[83] Rather than a controlling supreme being, though, Cherokees showed respect to multiple spiritual forces, brought oppositional powers into balance, built community solidarity, and created an opportunity to survive in a dangerous world.

• • • •

The Cherokees' world of course became even more dangerous with the arrival of smallpox. The virus produced a sickness like no other that their medical practitioners had dealt with before. Aboriginal diseases typically struck one individual at a time and produced lasting chronic symptoms. If they produced death, they did so after a quite lengthy period. Smallpox of course made multiple individuals ill in rapid succession and produced strange symptoms that led to a quick death for many. Passivity, however, does not characterize the response of medical practitioners to the disease.

Cherokees drew on their preexisting cosmological knowledge and explained outbreaks of smallpox as a consequence of disrespect shown to the spirit world. But which beings could have been so angry at the people to inflict something as deadly upon them as smallpox? The guardian spirits of the animals might on the surface provide a quick answer to this question, especially given the pivotal role they played in a Cherokee story about Little Deer inflicting harm on hunters who failed to seek forgiveness for slaying terrestrial prey. If so, this experience would be similar to that of the Natives of eastern Canada, as the historian Calvin Martin has discussed. Martin's thesis, however, has no obvious applicability to the Cherokees. First, epidemics were not a prerequisite for their involvement in trade with Europeans. Cherokee trading activities with the English as discussed in the previous chapter stemmed from material desires to acquire manufactured goods and the martial necessity of having guns in the increasingly violent world that European imperialism produced. Second, Cherokees did not necessarily have to give up their ritual protocol in killing deer in order to participate in the fur trade. The trade built on traditional masculine pursuits, which continued to be surrounded with spiritual activities well into the nineteenth century.

Finally, and more to the point, no evidence indicates that Cherokees ever blamed spiritual gamekeepers on epidemics of smallpox and other colonial germs they faced.[84]

Instead, Cherokees believed that a higher order of beings inflicted them with devastating new diseases due to human failure to mediate properly with the spirit world. The first glimpse of this conclusion comes with Longe's early eighteenth-century discussion with a Cherokee priest. The holy man spoke of an upper world ruled by a "great emperor," a being that likely did not have the supreme authority that the monotheistic Longe interpreted it as having but that nonetheless exercised great power over the day-to-day lives of humans. This great emperor—perhaps a singularization of the thunder spirits described in nineteenth-century ethnography—had a connection to the four winds, or what Longe rendered as "petty gods." Humans had to show proper respect to the various spirits on a daily basis by sacrificing meat of a newly killed deer to the fire. Respect also had to be shown through the multiple periodic rites that marked the Cherokees' annual calendar. Failure, according to the priest, "causes the anger of the great Uka or emperor, and he sets all these 4 petty gods against the earth to destroy the crops and brings a famine." Such misdeeds included "disobeying their kings and superiors, . . . misbelieving the priests and not obeying the doctoring and good counsel that they give them and debauching of men's wives and stealing and lying that causes bloodshed amongst neighbors."[85]

The priest particularly pointed to ill behavior regarding the Green Corn Ceremony. Longe related that the priest's duties included informing their followers that they must take special medicines and perform the Going-to-Water rite as part of the larger ceremony, for, if they did not, then the great emperor would send the four winds as "messengers either with war or sickness or some grievous famine to destroy . . . rebellious people."[86] Longe later added that lightning descended from the upper world and brought disease to disobedient people. "Whenever the thunder falls on trees they will not approach within 50 paces of it," the trader recorded in reference to his Cherokee commercial partners. "They say that the ground is dreadful where it falls, and if they fall by chance within such a bounds and the soles of their feet touch the ground that they will break [out] all with sores."[87]

That the "sickness" or "sores" that Longe's priest mentions represented smallpox of course cannot be determined with certainty, but
the English trader recorded this interesting explanation not long after
the Cherokees' most likely first experienced the disease in the late
1690s. Longe's account thus suggests his Native partners had incorporated epidemics into their cosmology as a consequence of a rupture
in the reciprocal relationship between humans and the spirit world,
particularly the thunders and winds.[88]

James Adair's more well-known account of the 1738–39 epidemic
in some ways is similar to Longe's, although Adair's is more flawed
due to its goal of proving that indigenous peoples of the Americas
descended from the Lost Tribe of Israel. Adair demonstrates how the
Cherokees believed the epidemic to be a consequence of their own
disrespect of the spirit world, but he put an Old Testament spin on
indigenous actions and beliefs. Cherokee priests had supposedly
blamed the adultery of their young people for bringing upon them
"divine anger." Medical practitioners, however, certainly believed
a deeper offense was involved. Cherokees had a different attitude
from their English contemporaries when it came to sex and marriage.
Married individuals could essentially divorce their partners and chose
another with little social stigma.[89] Instead of such sinful conduct,
Cherokee practitioners were more concerned with appeasing the
spirits believed to bring them good harvests. Adair's account hints
at this by reporting that the adulterous activities "broke down and
polluted many of the honest neighbors' bean-plots" and that such
actions "would cost a great deal of trouble to purify again."[90] Such
actions were considered taboo not because of the intercourse itself
but because human fluids—blood and semen—were seen as polluting.
The ceremonial rites that had previously been practiced to ensure a
good harvest in other words had been violated and such disrespect
represented egregious error that brought catastrophe.

Outside of Adair's passage on the 1738–39 epidemic, he indicates
a Cherokee belief that the thunders were responsible for smallpox.
In a separate section of his memoirs, he wrote:

> Nothing sounds bolder, or is more expressive, than the Cherokee name
> of thunder, *Eentaquàróske*. It points at the effects and report of the battles,

THE

H I S T O R Y

OF THE

AMERICAN INDIANS;

PARTICULARLY

Thofe NATIONS adjoining to the MISSISIPPI, EAST AND
WEST FLORIDA, GEORGIA, SOUTH AND
NORTH CAROLINA, AND VIRGINIA:

CONTAINING

An ACCOUNT of their ORIGIN, LANGUAGE, MANNERS, RELIGIOUS and
CIVIL CUSTOMS, LAWS, FORM of GOVERNMENT, PUNISHMENTS, CONDUCT in
WAR and DOMESTIC LIFE, their HABITS, DIET, AGRICULTURE, MANU-
FACTURES, DISEASES and METHOD of CURE, and other Particulars, fuffi-
cient to render it

A

COMPLETE INDIAN SYSTEM.

WITH

OBSERVATIONS on former HISTORIANS, the Conduct of our Colony
GOVERNORS, SUPERINTENDENTS, MISSIONARIES, &c.

ALSO

AN APPENDIX,

CONTAINING

A Defcription of the FLORIDAS, and the MISSISIPPI LANDS, with their PRODUC-
TIONS—The Benefits of colonifing GEORGIANA, and civilizing the INDIANS—
And the way to make all the Colonies more valuable to the Mother Country.

With a new MAP of the Country referred to in the Hiftory.

By JAMES ADAIR, Efquire,
A TRADER with the INDIANS, and Refident in their Country for Forty Years.

LONDON:
Printed for EDWARD and CHARLES DILLY, in the Poultry.
MDCCLXXV.

James Adair's *History of the American Indians* (1775). Adair's depiction of the Cherokees' experience with smallpox in 1738 provides one of the most detailed accounts
of how indigenous practitioners responded to smallpox, but his desire to prove
that American Indians descended from the Lost Tribe of Israel flaws the evidence
that his work supposedly provides to support the "virgin soil" thesis. (Courtesy Special Collections, Kenneth Spencer Research Library, University of Kansas)

which they imagine the holy people are fighting above. The smallpox, a foreign disease, no way connatural to their healthy climate, they call *Oonatàquará*, imagining it to proceed from the invisible darts of an angry fate, pointed against them, for their young people's vicious conduct.

Such a passage suggests that the disease came down like lightning from the upper world.[91] Adair also depicted the thunders' representation on earth—fire—as being directly responsible for terrible diseases. Referring to Natives of the Southeast in general, he wrote that during the Green Corn Ceremony if individuals did not extinguish their old fires during the event, then "the divine fire will bite them severely with bad diseases, sickness, and a great many other evils."[92] The thunders gifted fire to humans to take care of them, but if people disrespected the sacred flames, then they could expect disaster. Native priests therefore demanded that their followers carefully observe the "ancient law" that prescribed proper ritual performance. If carefully observed, Adair remarked, then "the holy fire will enable their prophets, the rain-makers, to procure them plentiful harvests, and give their war-leaders victory over their enemies—and by the communicative power of their holy things, health and prosperity are certain." The priests warned, however, that "on failure, they are to expect a great many extraordinary calamities, such as hunger, uncommon diseases, a subjection to witchcraft, and captivity and death by the hands of the hateful enemy in the woods."[93]

While Adair's and Longe's descriptions lead readers to the upper world, other evidence of how Cherokees explained epidemics, particularly the 1738–39 outbreak, seemingly brings one back down to earth. In September 1739, Gen. James Oglethorpe, the commander and governor of the new colony of Georgia, met with some Cherokee leaders and recorded different details about their recent experience with smallpox, details that implicated a group to which Adair belonged—traders from South Carolina. Cherokees claimed, as Oglethorpe's secretary recorded, that "the smallpox, and rum carried up last winter by the unlicensed traders had slain near 1000 warriors & hunters among them. . . . That thereupon the Indians complained they had been poisoned."[94] Oglethorpe sent a more detailed report later and while he omitted a reference to poisoning, he still indicated that

Cherokees held Carolinian traders responsible for the mortality they suffered over the past year. So much so that they "demanded justice from all the English, threatened revenge and sent to the French for assistance."[95] Evidently, the English managed to absolve themselves of the alleged crime. Records do not indicate retaliation against the traders, and Cherokees remained allied to the English.

Allegations that smallpox stemmed from poisoned rum nonetheless deserve closer scrutiny. Did Oglethorpe and Adair simply get two different stories? Or is there perhaps a connection between rum and transgressions against spirits of the upper world? On one hand, Oglethorpe's and Adair's information could have come from Cherokees belonging to different towns or divisions, in which multiple explanations existed. The Cherokee Nation after all consisted of dozens of independent towns with a variety of medical practitioners. Some towns may have believed that rum played a role; others may not. Some may have believed that sexual intercourse in the bean plots created the offense; others may have cited other infractions. On the other hand, rum may have played a role in causing the spirits of the upper world to become angry. In this case, witchcraft instead of poisoning best describes how Cherokees viewed the actions of Carolinian traders. Recall that Cherokees believed that the spirit of a substance—not the material itself—possessed the power to cure because it worked against the spirit that caused illness; similarly any ingredient that traders added to the rum would not in itself have caused harm but instead would have been a medium that called upon powerful beings to come and punish the intended victims. Cherokees, who had experience with alcohol for at least a few decades, considered it a spiritually powerful and potentially dangerous beverage. But, they did not necessarily always associate it with malevolency.[96] Instead, the traders' actions brought into Cherokee communities evil spirits that contaminated communal rites, perhaps those purification ceremonies to which Adair alludes in his account, causing vengeful spirits to punish the people with smallpox.[97]

Butrick's records give a more complete picture of how Cherokees came to conceptualize smallpox. As did Longe and Adair, the nineteenth-century missionary described Cherokee beliefs about epidemics as stemming from transgressions against upper world beings.

Butrick, however, learned from his informants that a specific spirit carried smallpox. "The small pox was called Kosvkv Askini, that is, a kind of devil always disposed to evil," Cherokees explained.[98] Kosvkv Askini appears to be a particularly malevolent entity, different from the variety of ordinary Nanehi who moved through each level of the cosmos. One of Butrick's informants referred to the smallpox spirits as "a kind of people" with the females being "about the color of a ripe chestnut burr" and "covered with fine prickles" and the males being "about the color of a ripe poke berry." The female began the infection by giving an individual who touched her "fine red pimples," while the male followed by touching the victim and occasioning "the black appearance which the disease afterwards assumed."[99] Kosvkv Askini furthermore only slept at midnight and roamed in "the large, plain paths" upon which people ordinarily traveled.[100] Still, these devil-like beings were the tools of larger entities. Butrick's informants told him they were "kept confined by the three Beings above, except when they let him loose to kill people in that manner." The particular upper world spirits remained unidentified, although they were likely the thunders, given the cosmic association of these powerful spirits with chaos and disorder. Whoever they were, they sent smallpox when "they were displeased with the people for their sins."[101] Rather than "sins" in a Judeo-Christian sense, Cherokees courted disaster when they did not keep their medicine strong and their relations with the spirit world reciprocal. In such cases, terrible epidemiological misfortune occurred, just as Longe discovered as early as the 1710s and as Adair alludes to in his published memoirs.

● ● ● ●

Explaining smallpox within their own cosmology was one way Cherokees responded to the disease. Coping with an ongoing epidemic, however, presented a very difficult set of circumstances. Unfortunately, James Adair's memoirs provided the only direct observation of Cherokee actions amid an actual epidemic, and the picture that it painted, at least on the surface, was not flattering. The English trader portrayed Cherokees as responding in a counterproductive and then fatalistic way. To stop the disease, medical practitioners had their patients "lie out of doors, day and night, with their breast frequently open to the night dews, to cool the fever: they were likewise afraid, that the diseased would otherwise pollute the house, and by that means, procure all their deaths." Adair lamented that medical practitioners did not apply "warm remedies" but instead "in every visit poured cold water on their naked breasts, sung their religious mystical songs . . . with a doleful tune, and shook a calabash with the pebble-stones, over the sick, using a great many frantic gestures." When the epidemic continued to spread, practitioners ordered their patients to take a sweat bath and then submerge themselves in the cold water of a stream. Such a treatment, according to Adair, was essentially a death sentence. He remarked that their "rivers being very cold in summer, by reason of the numberless springs, which pour from the hills and mountains—and the pores of their bodies being open to receive the cold, it rushing through the whole frame, they immediately expired." Failure to halt the epidemic led medical personnel to discard their paraphernalia and "a great many" even to kill themselves.[102]

Adair's negative description of Cherokee practitioners, however, is problematic in several ways. The trader showed no modern knowledge of medicine but instead echoed flawed assumptions about disease and the body that circulated at the time in Great Britain and her American colonies. Adair in particular condemned cold treatment based on the idea that smallpox was some kind of poison that had to be expelled from the body. Some European treatments called for cooling fevers, but others called for warm treatment. Sweating, it was believed, kept the body's pores open and allowed toxins to escape, but such therapy was counterproductive. English physicians did not reduce fever when necessary, and, to make matters worse, they often accompanied their warm treatment with toxic drugs and a combination of bleeding, vomiting, and purging to induce the body to expel toxins.[103] Adair himself did not show much confidence in European medicine at the time, claiming that English doctors "seldom failed of poisoning their weak patients by slow degrees" and remarking favorably on Native physicians, whose simple herbal remedies offered more comfort.[104] By incorporating a bias against the Cherokees' cold regimen, however, the trader unfairly painted a picture of their medicine as backward even for its own time. Cherokee practices in fact were no worse than what Europeans did and may have in fact been better. Smallpox in particular could cause a fever so high that coma, brain damage, and even death could result. Cooling a patient thus might have actually saved some lives. Exposure to frigid river water, to be sure, could have been detrimental since it may have induced cycles of chills and fevers that drove temperatures even higher than they were originally. Nevertheless, Cherokee practitioners were only inept in that they lived in a day and age before modern medicine, a judgment that applied as well to their European counterparts, perhaps even more so.

In addition to his flawed biological knowledge, Adair did not fully relate the meaning of what Cherokee practitioners were doing. They were undoubtedly conducting a Going-to-Water rite, a practice not merely intended as a therapy but instead as an appeal to the spirit world. Long Man's powers, Cherokees hoped, might take away the sickness and cleanse participants of the impurities—the evil spirits that had invaded their dreams and bodies—that would endanger ceremonial activities, including those involved in healing. The rite, moreover, was an effort to restore cosmic balance by paying reverence to the sacred winds that blew from the cardinal directions.

While Adair misconstrued much of what the Cherokees did, he does include one crucial bit of evidence that counters the view of Native ineptness: the seclusion of sick patients from their community. Adair described practitioners sending their patients outside of the village and into the fields because "they were . . . afraid, that the diseased would otherwise pollute the house, and by that means, procure all their deaths." Such actions almost certainly slowed the spread of the disease, and one might read this as evidence of an indigenous understanding of smallpox as contagious. But, seclusion held another purpose in the minds of medical practitioners and their followers. Smallpox symptoms resembled those of individuals ordinarily kept from their villages, especially during communal ceremonies. Blood outside of the body, which often resulted from bursting smallpox pustules, presented a powerful anomaly much as did menstruation, leading practitioners to fear that infected individuals would ruin their power to mediate with the spirit world. Thus, Cherokees, although not in accord with modern conceptions of communicable disease, employed a form of quarantine in their response to the 1738 epidemic, and they would strive to keep themselves away from wherever the disease was suspected of lurking throughout the remainder of the eighteenth century.

Cherokees did not have to learn this strategy of quarantine and avoidance from supposedly more modern Europeans either. Eighteenth-century Europeans, to be sure, understood the communicable nature of smallpox; they believed that contact with the poisons being emitted from an infected person could make another sick. Someone like Adair may have related this view to Cherokees early in the eighteenth century, and the trader himself may have encouraged his indigenous clients to employ quarantine; he took partial credit, for example, in saving Creeks from the full impact of a smallpox epidemic in 1749. As he traveled through their nation with a group of other traders and Choctaws, he learned that the upper Creek towns had become infected, declaring, "The smallpox . . . would have greatly depopulated them, if the officious advice of some among us, for all the other towns to cut off every kind of communication with them, on the penalty of death to any delinquent, had not been given and pursued." He claimed that Creeks "accordingly posted sentinels at proper places, with strict orders to kill [an individual coming from an infected town], as the most dangerous of all enemies: and these cautious measures produced the desired effect."[105]

Cherokees, nonetheless, had practiced forms of seclusion well before Europeans arrived, and oral tradition indicates that they adapted such practices to deal with deadly illnesses. Butrick's informants told him:

> Long ago the Indians were afflicted with some very awful diseases which do not now prevail. One of these differed from the smallpox, or yaws, yet occasioned dreadful sores in the flesh. When any one in a family was taken with that disorder the diseased person was removed, and had a hut, or tent, raised at a distance from any other habitation, and there lived alone. Then the priest was sent for to cleanse the dwelling just left by the diseased, as if some person had died in it. After this should any one touch the diseased, he would be unclean as if he had touched a dead body.[106]

Again, the Cherokees' main concern was keeping their medicine strong to preserve cosmic balance and show respect to the spirit world, but the practical benefits of such concern should not be ignored. Seclusion may not have completely eliminated smallpox from their villages, but the practice certainly slowed the progress of an epidemic and allowed for a continuation of tasks necessary for survival. One should also not presume that ill patients were abandoned. Secluded individuals still had food, water, and medicine taken to them.[107] There is no reason to believe then that Natives necessarily and universally delivered counterproductive therapies for smallpox. Cherokees had an approach to deadly diseases such as smallpox that were no worse and may have in fact been better than those practiced by Europeans during the colonial era.

• • • •

For Cherokee practitioners, fighting smallpox was not just a matter of treating infected individuals but also involved the employment of preventative medicine. They attempted to keep their respective communities free from harm by bringing countervailing forces into action against those beings that caused the epidemic and thereby restoring their communities' relations with a variety of spirits. Cherokees adhered to their traditional round of ceremonies as the first round of defense against epidemics; failure to do so would, as previously noted, produce dangerous consequences that potentially included diseases. Their initial experiences with colonial germs, though, led them to believe that their usual rites were not enough to maintain the needed reciprocity with the various beings that inhabited the cosmos, particularly when "a very mortal sickness" approached. Cherokees created two new rituals in such contingent situations. Both were modified forms of the Atohvna, with one generally referred to as a "physic dance," which was designed to protect against epidemic diseases in general, and the other referred to as a "smallpox ceremony," which focused specifically on the most dreaded of colonial germs.[108]

The smallpox ceremony represents a particularly novel response to *Variola* that most powerfully stands in opposition to the "virgin soil" thesis's notion of Native ineptness and passivity. Information on this interesting practice comes to us through the writings of Butrick. Cherokees told him that they conducted this ceremony when the "strange beings" that caused smallpox lurked near their communities. As with the Atohvna, a town's Beloved Men oversaw preparations and selected a head practitioner; the chosen spiritual leader gathered a selection of "herbs & roots" for a communal medicine pot; a group of seven chosen men carefully maintained the fire; the community consumed medicines; and the practitioner sacrificed a buck's tongue and performed divination. Butrick learned some key details on the smallpox ceremony that were not associated with its Atohvna antecedent, however. Such details further illustrate how Cherokees conceived of smallpox. The priest's assistants generated the ceremonial fire by rubbing two sticks of basswood together and kindled it with dry pieces of the same material obtained from the eastside of the tree and free of worms and rot. Why basswood? This tree, Cherokees explained to Mooney, was resistant to lightning and held great spiritual powers. Ordinarily Cherokee hunters tapped into those powers by wearing belts made of the tree's stringy bark so that they would not be struck by lightning while pursuing game.[109] Incorporation of this wood into the smallpox ceremony thus infused Cherokee medicine with spiritual powers capable of defeating the thunders' creations.

Cherokees called upon a variety of other spiritual powers to countervail those that caused smallpox. Unfortunately, Butrick's description of the ceremony does not reveal what those powers might have been. The missionary only refers to practitioners praying to Kvtsaka, an unidentified upper world being, to come and take smallpox away.[110] Other sources indicate that Kvtsaka may have had a connection with birds and that spirits of these avian creatures were best to deal with smallpox. During an epidemic in 1824, for example, a group of Cherokee schoolchildren prayed to a great eagle above to take away the evil spirit believed to be spreading smallpox at the time. In some sense, the eagle served as medium to the upper world, taking the children's prayers to great beings above.[111] In another sense, this giant bird must have been seen as the oppositional spiritual force to that which caused smallpox. Eagles swooped down from above and whisked away snakes, which like smallpox was one of the thunders' creations.

Kvtsaka may have been the name Cherokees gave for the mythic ancestor of eagles, or it may have been the name of another bird: the Great Buzzard whose wings slapped the earth in its primordial state giving rise to the mountains and valleys that characterized the Cherokee homeland. This being's descendants came to be seen as "a doctor among birds" because it consumed decayed flesh and yet remained healthy, giving it the appearance of being immune to contagious diseases. Faced with smallpox during the American Civil War, Cherokee practitioners in fact recommended a preventative treatment that required their patients to consume a small portion of buzzard flesh or to bathe in a soup with the bird being the main ingredient.[112] Such an innovation almost certainly represents a Cherokee belief that bird spirits could be called upon to do battle with beings that caused smallpox.

Regardless of whether bird spirits were invoked, the smallpox ceremony embodied one major feature that made it unique. Throughout the seven days that it lasted, participants had strict prohibitions on their movements. Because Kosvkv Askini roamed common paths and rested only for a short time at midnight, people could not safely travel. Individuals could only move from their town house to their dwellings to acquire food. If people had to leave the village, they left their towns only at midnight and traveled through the woods rather than main routes. During the first night, everyone stayed awake and observed the fire and communal medicine pot. They remained "still & solemn as if in the house of death or mourning." At sunrise, the priest prayed to the east and distributed the medicine to the community. Participants fasted until after noon. Butrick's informants in fact made no mention of any dancing, whipping of the town's buildings, or Going-to-Water as in other annual ceremonies. All slept in the town house during the nights, consumed medicine from the communal pot "as they pleased," and observed "peculiar stillness" throughout. An exception to the restriction on movement and travel occurred only on the morning of the sixth day, when male hunters ventured into the woods to kill deer and acquire the tongue of a buck for sacrifice.[113]

The smallpox ceremony ended with the usual sacrifice, divination, and meal but included other innovative features. On the seventh day, the priest approached the fire from the east, placed the deer's tongue

onto the coals, sprinkled old tobacco, and "prayed to know whether
that disease they feared would be kept away or not." With his assistants and the Beloved Men, the practitioner carefully observed the
tongue and smoke. Perhaps they watched for messages from the
thunders whether Kosvkv Askini would be called back to the western
sky. In any event, the priest made known the results of his divination and ordered the people to eat. Lastly, the Beloved Men gave a
participant some of the fire and instructed him or her to "keep it as
long as he or she might live, keeping it in a room by itself, not cooking
by it, nor lighting a torch by it, nor suffering a coal of it to be thrown
out, where it will be extinguished."[114] One of Butrick's informants
in fact had been given that honor. He in turn gave it to his mother,
who still retained it "in a certain room by itself" and guarded it just
as the practitioner had prescribed.[115] Presumably the fire could be
employed again to prepare medicines and send messages to upper
world spirits when smallpox spirits reappeared.

Cherokees almost certainly invented the smallpox ceremony during
the eighteenth century, with the most plausible window of time for
its creation being 1739 to 1752. Adair did not mention it in context
of the tragic epidemic he supposedly witnessed, while the English
first made note of an important individual known as "Smallpox Conjuror of Settico" in 1752 and referred to him several times thereafter.[116]
Circumstantial evidence suggests he was leading a ceremony to avoid
Variola, at least on one occasion. With the dreaded disease spreading
throughout the Carolina Piedmont in 1759 and afflicting the nearby
Catawbas, an English officer informed the governor of South Carolina
that Smallpox Conjuror of Settico was "conjuring every day."[117] Of
course, this interesting practitioner may have taken on many opportunities to mediate between his community and the spirit world, and
his activities at that time might have been related to warfare. In any
event, it is not surprising that eighteenth-century records give us
little to go on regarding the origins and practice of this innovative
ceremony. The rite calls for Cherokee villages to be shut off from the
outside world and for participants to maintain the strictest purity.
Outsiders would not have been welcomed. The smallpox ceremony's
cousin—the physic dance—did not completely escape the attention
of literate Europeans, however. Two different Englishmen on two
different occasions—one in 1759 and one in 1762—made reference

to the physic dance, thus giving further evidence that Cherokees had by the mid-eighteenth century made important innovations to their ceremonial inventory, innovations that they designed to restore proper respect to the spirit world and thus shelter them from colonialism's loathsome germs.[118]

If the creation of the smallpox ceremony is not enough to show Native agency in fighting smallpox, other evidence in the historical record certainly does. On numerous occasions during the eighteenth century, Cherokee leaders counseled their followers to avoid areas known or suspected to be harboring *Variola* or other nasty germs. Natives, for example, frequently found Charles Town to be teeming with disease, and when they sent delegations there, members sometimes died. In 1749, such concerns led both Cherokees and Creeks initially to reject Gov. James Glen's request that they come visit him. They sent their reason through an English messenger that they "beg leave to represent to your Excellency the ill consequences that attends the headmen going to Charles Town by sickness, that from time to time they have lost a great many headmen and some they have lost since your Excellency's time."[119] The Native leaders asked that the conference be held at Fort Moore, an outpost opposite Augusta on the Savannah River. Unfortunately, Glen remained unmoved and insisted that meetings occur in Charles Town. The respective Cherokee and Creek delegations arrived by September 6, 1749, and quickly sickened. Glen made English doctors available to them but many died, including noted Cherokees Yellow Bird and his wife as well as the prince of Tennessee's son and "Half Breed Johnie," the "Greatest Warrior of the Cherokee Nation." Several Creeks perished as well and went home with ill feelings toward the English.[120] Given the timing and location of infection, yellow fever was likely responsible for the outbreak, but its exact identity cannot be known. *Variola* more certainly affected a group of Cherokee travelers later in the same year. Then, a group set out for Charles Town but had to stop along the way as some became sick with what they claimed to have been smallpox. None reportedly died, and those who had been infected resumed their journey after recovering.[121]

The Cherokees' experience with traveling into or through disease-infested places left a lasting legacy. When Glen again called on Cherokees to meet him in the colonial capital in 1755, Connecorte or "Old

Hop" of Chota, one of the most influential spiritual leaders in Cherokee history, would not consent to sending a delegation. Connecorte's reason, one trader reported, "was that he had from time to time according to your Excellency's orders and desire sent down the best of his warriors to Charles Town, and that by reason of sickness they contracted there, or on their journey homewards, they had lost their lives." The trader further related Cherokee repugnance of seeing the bones of their deceased kinsmen that still remained visible along the path that connected them to the English settlements.[122] Another trader thought that Connecorte's explanation was an "excuse," but he did not fully consider how Cherokees perceived the potential threat that awaited them along the way into the colonial capital.[123] James Adair offered a different interpretation of this same event that puts it more into context of indigenous medicine. The Cherokees, he recorded, had a "fear of pollution" as they went to Charles Town. "They are distant from their own holy places, and holy things, where only they could perform their religious obsequies of their dead, and purify themselves according to law."[124] A journey into the colonial capital in other words would bring them into contact with ghosts of their unburied dead, jeopardize their relations with the spirit world, and invite further calamities.

On several other occasions in the eighteenth century—as the next two chapters will discuss—Cherokees kept away from places where they suspected smallpox to lurk. Such "common sense" advice came from spiritual leaders who had supposedly lost their credibility due to their inability to deal with colonial germs. Practitioners, moreover, did more than just give that one bit of common sense. They created and conducted smallpox ceremonies that offered a degree of protection as well. The rite functioned as a form of quarantine with villages shut off from the outside world and prohibitions on traveling in the open implemented. The smallpox ceremony in other words demonstrates that Cherokees had the ability and the desire to fight against the disease. That they had this desire might strike one as absurd to have to say—who after all would not want to avoid smallpox? But given the emphasis of the "virgin soil" thesis on Native passivity and fatalism, the statement must be made. From a larger perspective, smallpox ceremonies helped Cherokees make sense of epidemics within their own cosmological framework and build community solidarity amid colonialism's biological consequences.

• • • •

Practitioners thus obviously continued to play an important role within Cherokee communities after the 1738–39 epidemic. So, what does one make of Adair's report of a "great many" Cherokee practitioners committing suicide, an episode that the historian William McLoughlin reads as evidence for the disappearance of a "priestly hierarchy"? There appears to be a clear contradiction in the evidence. On one hand, it is hard to interpret what Adair wrote without concluding that a significant degree of declension occurred. On the other hand, Cherokee ethnography reveals impressive persistence of a medical tradition in which practitioners continued to be trained in sacred knowledge and conduct healing and prevention ceremonies even against smallpox and other diseases.

To sort out this contradiction, let us revisit Adair's account once again. One can never fully understand of course what went through the minds of those who killed themselves, but it was almost certainly not for the reason the English trader ascribed. They killed themselves, according to Adair, because they could not imagine themselves living with the scarring pock marks that smallpox produced: "Being naturally proud, they are always peeping into their looking glasses, and are never genteelly dressed, according to their mode, without carrying one hung over their shoulders: by which means, seeing themselves disfigured, without hope of regaining their former beauty."[125] Rather than vanity, Cherokee priests observed the horror going on around them and likely discovered terrible omens in their divination crystals. Fear for the future of their community's health must have led them to such drastic measures. They must have also feared for their own lives, not just from the disease but from families of the deceased, who would have suspected them of employing witchcraft. Lastly, priests may have believed that they had become possessed by the spirits of the dead because of a failure to perform funerary customs in a proper way. Cherokees dealt with death in a very careful way.

As Butrick recorded, each community had a practitioner—denoted in the missionary's records as a male—that specialized in mortuary rites. This individual buried corpses either in the dwellings in which they died or in the case of "a distinguished chief" in the council house. The practitioner worked alone, removed all of the deceased's belongings, by either burning or burying them, extinguished the old fire, cleansed the hearth, and then produced a new fire. He then prepared purifying medicines for the deceased's family and led them in a Going-to-Water rite. Family members donned new clothes and were considered unclean for four days.[126] Such funerary customs were difficult if not impossible during a major epidemic, leading to fears that vengeful spirits lingered about their community rather than going off to the Darkening Land.

If a mass suicide of practitioners on the scale Adair indicated occurred, those losses in addition to those who died from disease resulted in some medical knowledge going with them to their graves. Subsequent generations of Cherokees certainly lost some of their cultural inheritance due to colonial epidemics—that is not disputed. But reading Adair's passage as evidence of a linear declension of Native medicine is problematic. Take, for example, his statement that "all the magi and prophetic tribe broke their old consecrated physic-pots, and threw away all the other pretended holy things they had for physical use, imagining they had lost their divine power by being polluted."[127] What the English trader failed to mention, however, is the cultural context of these actions. Again, Butrick's records sheds light on what practitioners must have been doing with an informant telling him, "If one, lost a patient, he threw away all the medicine like what he had used in that case, and used no more of it till it came new another year." The practitioner ceased his activities until the first new moon. At that time, he purified himself by consuming an emetic made of special roots and by pouring the medicine on a heated rock and bathing his hands in the steam that arose. Thereafter, the practitioner returned to healing and ceremonial practices.[128] Adair's omission then obscures a dynamic element of Cherokee medicine.

The disappearance of a hereditary priesthood due to their failure to deal with colonial germs also does not follow from the available evidence. In making this assertion, McLoughlin conflates Adair's account of the 1738–39 epidemic with a Cherokee legend of the Ani-Kutani. In the nineteenth century, Cherokees remembered them as an elite group who oversaw communal rituals, recited the nation's migration story, and spoke in a ceremonial language that common people did not understand. At some unspecified point, the Ani-Kutani took advantage of their privileged position, antagonized ordinary people, and suffered their downfall. The two distinct sources of this legend, however, differ in what happened to this priesthood. In 1809 the visiting Mohawk John Norton discussed this priesthood with a Cherokee speaker who told him that the Ani-Kutani indulged in unspecified "wickedness" and "vices" and were consequently "put to death where ever they were found."[129] Norton's account existed only in manuscript form until published in 1970. The second source—that of Charles Hicks—became more widely distributed. Hicks revealed the legend to the Tennessee historian Judge John Haywood, who published it in a truncated form in his 1823 *Natural and Aboriginal History of Tennessee*, and then in 1826 Hicks related a more detailed account to his fellow countryman John Ross.[130] Ross relayed the account to various others, including Dr. J. B. Evans, who was the main source for a version published in 1866.[131] Hicks's account offers more specifics than Norton's about the priesthood's downfall and ultimate fate. The priests allegedly demanded the wife of a young hunter, whose brother was a respected civil leader. The two men subsequently killed the priests, triggering others to do the same to individuals who belonged to the lofty order. Some Ani-Kutani escaped, yet they never retained their exalted role and instead devolved into less esteemed medical practitioners.

Neither of the two original accounts mentions anything about a failure to deal with new diseases. Disease only came into the story through the work of James Mooney and not the way McLoughlin suggests. Mooney had read the published versions of the legend, asked his informants about it, and learned that the Cherokees who spoke to him knew "so little" about the Ani-Kutani "that their very identity is now a matter of dispute." The anthropologist did add that his informants with "more authority, claim that they were a clan or society in the tribe and were destroyed long ago by pestilence or other calamity."[132] Only through a shaky inference then could one deduce that Cherokees had assassinated a hereditary priesthood due to a failure of their medicine amid colonialism's biological consequences. If disease had anything to do with their downfall, it most likely had decimated their ranks to the extent that they stopped functioning as a coherent order of practitioners. Even in this event, Cherokee medicine obviously continued; elders still trained their younger kinsmen in the sacred arts of healing and other medical rites; practitioners still treated patients and employed preventative strategies for the protection of their people; and by many accounts "conjurors" played a prominent leadership role through most of the eighteenth century.

Who then were the Ani-Kutani? The contemporary anthropologist Raymond Fogelson offers the best explanation. He argues that the legend did not have a basis in any one particular event in the past. Instead, the legend was a dramatic story that reflected two major elements. First, it epitomized the fundamental tensions between hierarchy and egalitarianism that characterized Cherokee life.[133] The legend in other words served as a useful check on the powers of those trained in sacred knowledge and helped maintain the Cherokees' decentralized leadership structure in which the more secular authority in the form of Ukas, Ravens, Beloved Men, and Beloved Women was balanced against the more sacred authority of the priests. Second, Fogelson suggests that the story reflected Cherokee efforts to comprehend the decline of "an elaborated priesthood." This decline, which he characterizes as "drastic" yet "gradual," occurred over the course of the eighteenth century as Cherokees lost power over their lives due to colonialism. Practitioners in other words lost significant status and influence due to a number of factors but did not disappear entirely.

• • • •

The analysis offered in this chapter and those to follow supports Fogelson's argument. The authority of practitioners did not collapse with a single event. The 1738–39 epidemic in particular did not represent an end of efforts to fight smallpox but an episode of an ongoing struggle against colonial germs, a struggle in which Cherokees did not give up on their medicine and in which their followers did not give up on their practitioners. The Ani-Kutani legend should not distract from the more important story. Natives responded actively and creatively to the biological consequences of colonialism. The smallpox ceremony provides telling evidence that Native medical practitioners did not always do as prevailing historiographical interpretations would have them do: fail to explain what was happening, refuse to deal with colonial germs, and decline in status and authority among their people. By explaining epidemics the way they did, sticking to aboriginal practices of seclusion, and creating new rituals, practitioners both reinforced Cherokee cosmology and built community solidarity amid potential for calamity. From a practical standpoint, they helped save lives. They counseled against traveling into disease-ridden settlements, while the smallpox ceremonies they conducted closed villages off against the outside world and helped curtail the spread of contagion. Rather than passivity then, Cherokees took actions that enhanced their ability to culturally and physical survive in a world increasingly filled with colonial germs.

The Natives' world, however, was becoming increasingly hazardous as the eighteenth century progressed. A growing Euro-American presence near Cherokees weakened their ability to control their exposure to introduced diseases. As the next two chapters reveal, war and all its malignant consequences bore down especially hard on the Cherokee people over the last half of the eighteenth century. The smallpox ceremony and avoidance strategies could not and did not always protect them, but this failure was not something inherent in their medicine. In this realm, Cherokee practitioners were much more capable of dealing with colonialism's most dreaded disease than one mere anecdote in the trader James Adair's memoir suggests and more than contemporary scholars have concluded.

CHAPTER 3

WAR

In early 1760, Lord Jeffery Amherst—the commander in chief of British forces in North America—wanted the Cherokee Nation destroyed, and smallpox appeared poised to do the job for him. Cherokees had been Britain's most important indigenous partner in their ongoing conflict with the French, but that changed in the latter stages of the conflict commonly known as the French and Indian War or, more appropriately, the Seven Years' War in North America (1754–60). During the spring and summer of 1758, settlers murdered at least thirty Cherokee men on their way back from helping the British defeat the French in the Ohio Valley, and when the British failed to make proper satisfaction, Cherokees decided to exact vengeance and escalated what became known as the Anglo-Cherokee War (1759–61). Warriors descended on colonists in the southern backcountry in spring of 1759. South Carolina governor William Henry Lyttelton subsequently had his colony declare war in October, and he personally led militia forces to southern Appalachia. Smallpox beat him there. The virus had been spreading through the Piedmont for several months and reached the eastern most Cherokee town of Keowee by December. Lyttelton's troops too became infected, leaving the governor no choice but to abandon his invasion and call upon Amherst for help. Amherst ordered troops under Col. Archibald Montgomery to the south to take care of the situation. "You will . . . punish the Indians for this infamous breach of the peace they had so lately made," Amherst ordered Montgomery, "in such manner that His Majesty's subjects may hereafter enjoy their possessions without any dread of these barbarous and inhuman savages."[1] To Lyttelton, Amherst responded that "it remains for us now to chastise their insolence, and endeavor to reduce them so low, that they may never more be able to be guilty of the like again."[2] Meanwhile, the Cherokees struggled to prevent the most devastating colonial germ from causing widespread damage.

Amherst, to be sure, did not instruct Montgomery to deliberately infect Britain's Native adversaries with smallpox as he would do some three years later. In 1763, with the Lenapes, Shawnees, Ottawas, and others besieging Fort Pitt during what is most often called Pontiac's War, the commander infamously asked Col. Henry Bouquet: "Could it not be contrived to send the *smallpox* among those disaffected tribes of Indians? We must, on this occasion, use every stratagem in our power to reduce them?"[3] Both Amherst and Bouquet had previously learned the disease had broken out among the British in the fort and that the infected had been quarantined in a hospital at the outpost. Bouquet answered positively to his superior's question, writing, "I will try to inoculate the Indians by means of blankets that may fall in their hands."[4] Amherst then gave further approval: "You will do well to try to inoculate the *Indians* by means of blankets as well as to try every other method, that can serve to extirpate this execrable race."[5] Whether Bouquet ever carried out what Amherst suggested is unknown, but it turns out he may not have needed to. Officers inside of Fort Pitt enacted what their commanders had contemplated well before the colonel's arrival on August 10. On June 24 two Lenape leaders visited the fort to negotiate a peace and then returned to their people with deadly gifts. "Out of our regard to them we gave them two blankets and an handkerchief out of the smallpox hospital," Capt. William Trent recorded in his journal.[6] Later, Fort Pitt's commander Simon Ecuyer certified a reimbursement for the "sundries got to replace in kind those which were taken from people in the hospital to convey the smallpox to the Indians."[7] Over one year later, the account reached the desk of Gen. Thomas Gage, who had by then replaced Amherst as supreme commander. Gage endorsed the reimbursement.[8]

As the evidence relating to Fort Pitt in 1763 clearly shows, Europeans at least on one occasion contemplated, conducted, and approved the use of smallpox as a weapon against indigenous peoples. But how often did this happen? Scholars disagree. Earlier historians have generally treated the Fort Pitt incident as an isolated and atypical event. The nineteenth-century historian Francis Parkman first brought the Amherst-Bouquet correspondence to light. He characterized Amherst's original question as an aberration, one brought on by a "despicable enemy" who "pushed him to such straits" that he conceived of the "detestable suggestion."[9] Today, the roles of victims and victimizers have been reversed in public discourse, and Amherst has come to represent what one scholar calls "a shorthand censure of Europeans' treatment of native people." Assertions that the Fort Pitt incident typifies widespread and effective uses of smallpox are pervasive.[10] The most widely cited expert on the subject, Elizabeth Fenn, has given such beliefs persuasive scholarly support. She acknowledges that except for the Fort Pitt incident documented cases for germ warfare have not and likely cannot be found, but she opens her readers up to the possibility of more examples and indicates why it would be the case that written proof for these does not exist. She emphasizes that smallpox's communicable nature and its ability to spread through contaminated objects were well understood before Amherst penned his infamous question. Accusations of its use as a weapon were also common in eighteenth-century America, and such actions would not have been unprecedented as the use of disease and poison against enemies had occurred in European warfare well before 1763. Still, Europeans considered biological warfare beyond the pale of civilized behavior, would not want the stigma of being its perpetrators, and would have refrained from producing incriminating documents. This broader context, Fenn argues, suggests that "actual incidents may have occurred more frequently than scholars have previously acknowledged."[11] Some scholars, though, remain unconvinced and maintain that Amherst's correspondence was mere musing and what happened at Fort Pitt remains a singular event.[12]

While an interesting debate, the extent to which colonizers used smallpox as a weapon against indigenous peoples distracts from what can be concluded with certainty yet still remains obscured by the "virgin soil" thesis. Germs and warfare, as can be seen in the Anglo-Cherokee War, were intimately connected. A few years prior to the Fort Pitt incident, Amherst oversaw a campaign that resulted in his

Cherokee adversaries suffering from smallpox, not as a result of a deliberate effort to convey the germ to them but instead as a result of a scorched-earth campaign that deprived Natives of sustenance, created a mass of refugees, and curtailed them from taking effective measures to inhibit infections. Amherst's orders in other words were neither less brutal nor less epidemiologically significant than those he would make years later. His prosecution of the war against the Cherokees in fact demonstrates the more prevalent way in which human agency, rather than the supposed weakness of Native bodies, shaped indigenous experience with *Variola*.

• • • •

By the mid-1750s, the Cherokees should have been poised to recover from colonialism's past traumas. Their war with the Creeks, which the English continually stoked, terminated in 1753, their horticultural production remained relatively stable, many individuals had acquired immunity to smallpox by surviving the 1738–39 epidemic, and medical practitioners had developed ways to protect their people from exposure to *Variola* and other contagious diseases. Keeping their children safe and fostering their development into adults of reproductive age would indeed be essential for population recovery. The Seven Years' War, however, spawned another great smallpox epidemic and engulfed indigenous peoples throughout eastern North America in a maelstrom of violence, infection, and mortality.

As the British and French empires mobilized their armies, navies, and Native allies in a contest for the continent, the smallpox virus circulated over a vast space through the duration of the conflict. The epidemic began during the summer of 1755 within the St. Lawrence Valley, when *Variola* afflicted French settlements and Catholic Indian missions.[13] The disease spread south and west striking French soldiers at Fort Niagara and the Senecas, the westernmost and most anti-English member of the Iroquois Confederacy.[14] *Variola* persisted around Fort Niagara into 1756.[15] The British too suffered. A large body of King George II's troops arrived in Philadelphia in fall of 1756 already suffering from smallpox.[16] The disease then became rampant throughout Pennsylvania and persisted through 1757.[17] A party of pro-English

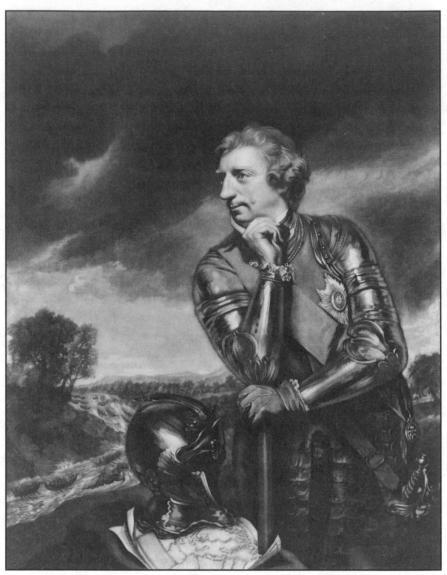

Sir Jeffery Amherst, engraving by James Watson (1766). Famous in his lifetime as Great Britain's hero who conquered Canada and infamous today as the villain who asked his subordinate to deliver smallpox blankets to indigenous peoples, Amherst ordered a brutal scorched-earth campaign against the Cherokee Nation in 1760 and 1761—an action that has been vastly overshadowed by his legacy as a perpetrator of biological warfare at Fort Pitt in 1763. (Courtesy of the Library of Congress, Prints and Photographs Division, LC-USz62–45182)

Iroquois and their confederates negotiating with the English at Lancaster came down with the dreaded germ in May. Fourteen died and their infected kinsmen then carried it back to the upper Susquehanna and Mohawk Valleys where it lingered through the summer.[18] France's western allies tumbled into this swirling storm of smallpox when large numbers of them entered the war during the summer of 1757. Nearly one thousand warriors, some from as far west as Iowa, joined the French in their 1757 offensive. With the aid of these warriors, General Montcalm laid siege on Fort William Henry on Lake George in New York and forced the British to surrender on August 8, 1757. Participation, though, led to infection. Warriors carried *Variola* back to their Great Lakes villages, where it made "great ravages." An untold number of Potawatomies, Ottawas, Menominees, and others perished during the fall and winter of 1757 and 1758.[19]

Amid this great smallpox epidemic, disease became a political issue in both France's and Britain's efforts to mobilize their respective native allies. During the summer of 1756, for example, France's western allies learned that smallpox lurked around French forts to the east, and they refused to go to these rendezvous points for military offensives against the English.[20] When the epidemic seemed to abate in 1757, they took part in Montcalm's offensive against Fort William Henry but their subsequent infection required France to undertake difficult negotiations. In January 1758 an officer reported from Fort Detroit that "the Indians who came to the army during the last campaign have lost many people from smallpox. Their custom in such a case is to say that the nation which called upon them has given them bad medicine." In an effort to exonerate themselves from what were in essence accusations of witchcraft, the French had to offer gifts to those who lost loved ones. "It is a mourning which will cost the king dearly," the Detroit officer remarked.[21] The French attempted to turn the blame on their imperial adversaries and had some success. An English prisoner among the Potawatomies recalled that his captors lost a "great Number" during and after returning from Fort William Henry and blamed the English for "poisoning the rum & giving them the smallpox."[22]

Insinuations of such malevolence persisted in Native oral history. A nineteenth-century Ottawa account claims that the smallpox epidemic originated with a particular item that "was sold to them" in Montreal. Specifically, the warriors carried home with them a tin box that contained a series of smaller tin boxes. In the smallest of the containers, "they found nothing but moldy particles." A "great many" examined the odd material and "pretty soon burst out a terrible sickness among them."[23] The Ottawas remembered it as horrific experience with "Lodge after lodge totally vacated—nothing but dead bodies lying here and there in their lodges—entire families being swept off with the ravages of this terrible disease." While the French would seem to bear responsibility for this catastrophe, the account did not indicate who sold them the deadly goods. Some Natives, moreover, specifically placed responsibility with the English with a nineteenth-century Ottawa man recounting, "This wholesale murder . . . by this terrible disease sent by the British people was actuated through hatred, and expressly to kill off the Ottawas and Chippewas because they were friends of the French Government or French King."[24]

Disease also became a political issue in the South. There, the French tried to lure the Cherokees away from their friendship with the British by making accusations of biological warfare. In the fall of 1756, a delegation of Overhills visited French officials at Fort Toulouse on the upper Alabama River and then at New Orleans. Fort Toulouse's commander told the delegation's leader, the Mankiller of Great Tellico, that he should not be fooled by the governor of South Carolina, who "gave him a fine red coat, but that was not all, for that coat had always something in it that would do his business for him before he could get home." The business was death by disease. The commander of Fort Toulouse further charged that "the Carolina People had conjurors amongst them that could send up different bundles of sickness to their nation from which proceeds the decrease of their people."[25] The French added another accusation that the English deliberately poisoned their allies. French officers claimed that the food they provided visiting Native emissaries was always "good and wholesome," but the governor of South Carolina gave his Native visitors food that "was mixed with something that was sure to kill some of them before they returned to their Nation." Aware that Cherokees and Creeks had occasionally perished on their way back from Charles Town, the French officers charged "that the Governor of Charles Town had killed so many of their people in that manner that his arms and hands must needs be all stained with blood."[26] At New Orleans, Governor Louis Billouart, Chevalier de Kerlérec, took his opportunity at persuading Cherokees to turn away from the malevolent British. "Whenever they [the Cherokees] went to the Governor of Carolina," Kerlérec charged, "he mixed their drink and victuals with something that killed them, but there were many hundreds of Indians come to him, and always went away well satisfied. That the Governor of Carolina was a rogue and only sent for them that he might be the cause of their death." The French governor then urged them to turn on the British.[27]

Such accusations did not work. Some Cherokees certainly retained suspicions about the English but the larger part of the nation remained wary of the French and instead gave essential assistance to Great Britain during the Seven Years' War. For their part, the French had given Cherokees little reason to trust them. King Louis XV's empire provided little in the way of gifts that could have established an alliance, while the British came through with measures that convinced a sizeable number of Cherokee warriors to enter the conflict. South Carolina's construction of Fort Loudoun on the Little Tennessee River among the Overhill Towns appears to have triggered Cherokee participation in the conflict. The Cherokees had called for this fort for some time, believing it would deter attacks on them by French-allied tribes to the north and west, and in the event of such attacks it would serve as a safe haven for their women and children.[28] Cherokee women also valued the fort for the market it provided for their agricultural products, while men appreciated the outpost for the blacksmith who repaired their guns.[29] After Loudoun's completion in late 1756, several hundred warriors tracked north to battle the Lenapes, Shawnees, Ottawas, and other French-allied tribes, whose raids had produced much death and suffering for British settlers in the mid-Atlantic back-country.[30] Cherokee warriors inflicted a series of punishing blows on France's native allies, while diplomats began negotiations for a pro-English alliance with the Six Nations. In the spring of 1758, hundreds more Cherokees went north to assist British general John Forbes in his expedition to Fort Duquesne. Perhaps as many as 1,200 Cherokee warriors made their way into Pennsylvania. Their presence along with their alliance with the Six Nations turned the tide of the war in the Ohio Valley. The Lenapes had suffered so much that they became amenable to a peace treaty, which led the French to abandon Fort Duquesne and the British to build Fort Pitt.[31]

While Cherokees assisted the British in scoring an important victory, they encountered the ongoing smallpox epidemic. *Variola* circulated among General Forbes's troops and may have played a role in leading Cherokees to quickly return home instead of remaining with the British through the duration of the campaign against Fort Duquesne. After peaking in early May, the number of Cherokee warriors dwindled to a mere two hundred by early June. There were multiple reasons for this exodus: the British were ill prepared to provide supplies, food, and gifts that they had promised; British officers generally treated Natives, particularly their war leaders, with contempt; Forbes appeared to be long delayed in assembling his troops; and news arrived that Virginians had murdered some of their countrymen.[32] Smallpox's presence in the northern theater, however, may have added to the Cherokees' general discontent without the British realizing it. On May 24, for example, news that the disease broke out among troops at Maryland's Fort Frederick had reached Winchester, Virginia, where a number of Cherokees had gathered. On the same day, forty Cherokees left for home and the remainder refused to go farther north.[33] "I am not able to devise what this humor of the Indians proceeds from," one British officer puzzled.[34] One cannot conclusively prove, of course, that smallpox drove the warriors away but the circumstances do suggest that potential infection added to all the other problems that the English faced in keeping Cherokees involved in the campaign.

For those who remained in the north, smallpox proved to be a danger. The disease persisted at Fort Frederick, spread to nearby Fort Cumberland, and then ultimately to Winchester.[35] There it had infected at least two of the Cherokees who remained willing to stay and fight against the French. These two individuals contracted the disease before setting out for a British camp in Pennsylvania, commanded by none other than Col. Henry Bouquet. One arrived with visible symptoms and the other became terribly ill just days after.[36] Unlike in 1763, it was in the colonel's interest to keep smallpox from spreading, certainly among his own troops, but also among Cherokees whom he wanted to keep as scouts for Forbes's advance to the Ohio. Bouquet had the infected warriors quarantined and put under the care of a British doctor. "This trifle is for them the greatest mark of confidence," he remarked.[37] Still, he maintained contempt for Natives. Bouquet continually railed against his indigenous allies, especially for their demands for presents and unwillingness to follow orders. He charged, "It is a great humiliation for us to be obliged to suffer the repeated insolence of such rascals. I think it would be easier to make Indians of our white men than to coax that damned tawny race."[38] Bouquet's disdain certainly did not bode well for British efforts to retain the help of the Cherokees. Neither did the ongoing smallpox epidemic and the terribly ill health that plagued Forbes's troops. Cherokees continued to trickle away from the British over the summer. By mid-September, with his drive to Fort Duquesne well behind schedule, General Forbes would have virtually no Native auxiliaries to scout ahead of his advance forces as they came within striking distance of Fort Duquesne, unless more Cherokees from their nation arrived.

Back in southern Appalachia, potential infection factored into Cherokee decisions to curtail their support of the British. Conflict between Virginians and Cherokees, to be sure, proved most consequential in their refusal to offer the British any more aid, but the specter of disease added to the growing rift. Warriors belonging to the Middle Town of Jore, for example, had been warned by a Carolinian trader "not to mind the talks of the warriors that came from Virginia and Carolina, but to remember how many of your people has died going to Carolina and to the assistance of the white people at different times, and that their bones lay white upon the road, and if you go with these warriors to Virginia, it's so far that you will die or be killed for not a man of you will ever return."[39] Leaders from Jore and nearby Watagi hesitated in sending warriors to the north and politely informed Governor Lyttelton that they would not go to Charles Town for further negotiations, although indicating that they did not subscribe to French insinuations that English governors practiced bad medicine. "The hot Weather is coming on," they claimed. "We lost a great many of our people by sickness going down in the summer; we don't blame you nor no other governor for that." They demurred until leaders of Chota, the mother town of the Overhills and the most important political center of the nation at the time, had a chance to fully consider the situation.[40]

Chota's medical practitioners indeed determined the situation unsafe for Cherokee warriors to go north, at least during the summer. In late June, the English recruitment officer George Turner received an answer from the Overhills that "it was the opinion of the conjurors that there would be much sickness and death attend them, and that they refused to go till fall." Turner became so worried that his superiors would believe him derelict in his duties that he immediately dictated a statement detailing the Cherokees' refusal. Eight Overhill leaders— including one just named as "Conjuror"—made their marks on the document while two interpreters, the commander of Fort Loudoun, and three other Englishmen signed it.[41] The next day Turner reported privately in a letter that practitioners "trumped up" the story of their people's predicted sickness, but in another letter he added details that revealed an acute awareness among Cherokees of the growing demographic disparities that colonialism had wrought.[42] Attakullakulla, one of the most influential Overhill leaders, stated his people "did not love to lose their young men" and "that they may not recruit their people as the whites did, who were like leaves of the trees."[43] Attakullakulla spoke with a degree of authority on this disparity. He had been to England as a young man back in 1730, saw the vast population there, and then came back to see the Cherokee Nation suffer population losses from smallpox in 1738–39 and their ongoing war with the Creeks. Turner continued to pressure Attakullakulla to lead his men into battle but received a promise to go only when the weather cooled. It was within that context that the leader explained that "they never undertook anything of consequence" without first consulting with "their conjurers."[44] Thus, only foolish warriors would go north in the heat of the summer, at a time that the medicine practitioner predicted "a pestilential distemper" would strike them and cause "a great many" to die.[45] Attakullakulla indeed waited until after the second Green Corn Ceremony to finally make good on his promise that he would go north. He arrived at Forbes's camp in Pennsylvania on

October 15 with a mere thirty warriors to assist the British in their final push toward Fort Duquesne.

Was smallpox the "pestilential distemper" that Cherokee practitioners worried about? The evidence to answer this question is mixed. On one hand, Cherokees expressed their fears in reference to traveling during the summer, leading one to conclude that they were not particularly concerned with smallpox but rather a disease like the one that their diplomats suffered so severely from while visiting Charles Town in 1749. On the other hand, circumstances would seem to indicate that smallpox was also on their minds. Recall that the British began to report the dreaded disease among their troops in the mid-Atlantic backcountry on May 24, while Turner received his rebuke by June 22. Warriors who returned home between the two dates possibly brought news of smallpox without bringing the virus itself as no outbreak appears to have occurred among the Cherokees throughout the summer. That was not the case for a nearby settlement of Chickasaws, who lived near the trading center of Augusta, Georgia. The virus reached them from an unknown source by June 10 and caused several deaths.[46] Governor Lyttelton enacted a quarantine of Augusta, but such orders did not keep the disease contained. Within weeks it spread among plantations in Georgia and South Carolina.[47] Since Augusta served as a point of departure for several unlicensed traders trafficking in rum, news of smallpox probably spread from there to southern Appalachian villages.[48] Medical practitioners likely incorporated such information into their prognostications.

Cherokees thus had much to worry about by the end of 1758. The emerging conflict with backcountry settlers and the closeness of colonial germs posed great challenges. During such ominous times, practitioners performed their regular cycle of ceremonies and turned to their innovative disease avoidance rites. The Reverend William Richardson observed this first hand when he arrived at Chota in January 1759. He lamented the power of the "conjurers" and recorded that "they have these few days been preparing a physic which they say will drive away all their disorders & the man to whose care it was committed has been every night and morning going round the town house hollowing & crying & frequently in the day to the great

man above for a blessing on the physic, as they say."[49] Richardson
had hoped to make converts, but the targets of his missionary zeal
remained wedded to their own beliefs, found the visitor to be a
nuisance, and told him to leave.[50] More specifically, practitioners
strove to keep their medicine strong by paying reverence to multiple spiritual beings, building community solidarity, and working to
restore cosmic balance.

• • • •

When the Cherokees went to war in the North, smallpox stayed away
from their nation in the South. When the war came to them, their
nation sat squarely on the path of the most destructive of colonial
germs. By the end of 1758, more than thirty Cherokee warriors lay dead
on the path to and from Winchester, Virginia. Settlers attacked these
Cherokees for a variety of reasons, including genuinely mistaking
them for French-allied Shawnees, retaliating for real and alleged rob-
beries, and cynically cashing in on bounties for enemy scalps without making efforts to distinguish between Native friends and foes.
Cherokees defended themselves at times as well, leaving settlers dead
and their families determined to take vengeance. Cool heads prevailed
among the Cherokees for the remainder of 1758 and into the first part
of 1759. Their leaders hoped that the British would make amends
by giving gifts to cover the dead and sorrowful talks that would
restore the alliance that they had long had. By April, however, the
colonial governors of Virginia and South Carolina had yet to assuage
the Cherokees, and kinsmen of the slain warriors avenged their losses.
Acting largely independent of other towns, Settico sent war parties
upon settlers in North Carolina. This town had suffered the most
deaths and took a like number of lives from British settlements.
Governor Lyttelton of South Carolina implemented a trade embargo
on Settico and demanded that the warriors who had perpetrated
the raids be surrendered to him for punishment. The governor was
rejected, and in August parties from the Lower Towns, who also lost
kinsmen on the path to Virginia, exacted their vengeance. Lyttelton
then extended the trade embargo onto all Cherokee towns, made
hostages of twenty-eight men from the indigenous nation who had

traveled to Charles Town to negotiate a settlement, and mobilized South Carolina's militia for a march to the southern Appalachians. In November, his troops set out for their expedition with the prisoners and their families in tow. The governor hoped that with this display of force he could use the hostages as a bargaining chip to coerce Cherokees to surrender to him the twenty-four men most responsible for raids on setters.[51]

Lyttelton's intentions were more modest than the advice he received from other British officials. Busy planning for the conquest of Canada, Lord Jeffery Amherst admitted he had little experience with indigenous peoples and did not want to get involved in affairs in the South. The general instead gave encouragement from afar. Referring to the Cherokees as "barbarians" and "dastardly scoundrels," he urged South Carolinians to "punish their outrages" so that "they will stand in greater awe of them," thus making it unnecessary to divert the king's forces. "I find that the only way to deal with them is to reward or punish them according to their deserts," he concluded without detailing what exactly punishment would involve.[52] North Carolina's governor Arthur Dobbs offered more concrete suggestions about what to do with the Cherokees. His colony bore the brunt of Native reprisals and he called for the indigenous nation to be wiped off the map. Dobbs quipped to Lyttelton, "In my opinion we should be proclaimed to enter their country at once burn their towns, take them their wives & children and sell them in the islands for slaves and give a premium of £10 for every person above 10 years of age but nothing for scalps unless killed in action."[53] Governor Lyttelton, who did not share Dobbs's genocidal hopes, proclaimed that the "object should rather be to reduce that people to proper submission than to depopulate them more than needed." His colony had long capitalized on a lucrative deerskin trade with Cherokees, and he still saw the indigenous nation as a "useful barrier for us against the French." The governor, however, stated he would proceed with "vigor," if they refused to accede to his demands.[54]

Before Lyttelton's troops could act with "vigor," they had to navigate their way through the smallpox epidemic that then ravaged Native and non-Native residents of the southern backcountry. *Variola* continued to circulate among Natives and settler communities of the Carolina Piedmont. It bore down particularly hard on the Catawbas. The Reverend Richardson indicated that the disease caused Natives to flee into the woods, where "great numbers" died.[55] Such high death tolls indicate that it had been some time since the Catawbas last experience with the disease and that measles may have been at work as well. Both diseases had been reported at Winchester, Virginia, in June, and it was from there that the Catawbas reported as having become infected.[56] Lyttelton had wanted the Catawbas to join him in his expedition against the Cherokees, but their leader, King Hagler, could only promise the governor that he would try "to keep our people together as much as possible to prevent the Disorder from spreading amongst ye white people until our people get well."[57] Catawbas had another incentive to retreat to their towns. They feared that settlers might mistake them for Cherokees and kill them. Such efforts only escalated infections among the Catawbas and prolonged the epidemic.[58] Caught between warring Carolinians and Cherokees and stricken with deadly germs, their population plummeted. The *South Carolina Gazette* reported that "near one half" of the Catawbas had perished.[59]

By November 11, Cherokees knew that both smallpox and Lyttelton's troops were near. Lower Town leaders learned "that most of the head men and warriors of the Catawbas were carried off by the smallpox" yet at the same time they feared that the intent of South Carolina's army "was to destroy all their towns and make captives of their women & children." In response, Cherokees called their hunters in, while the women prepared "to take to the hills with their children." Richard Coytmore, the commander of Fort Prince George, believed that the Lower Cherokees would abandon their towns.[60] James Adair recalled Cherokee reactions a little differently. He claimed the Lower Towns considered sending their warriors against Lyttelton's troops, but they concluded that the army's approach so near the onset of winter signaled its "innocent intentions" and they feared that if they did act offensively against the British they would not have the support of other divisions of their nation. "Their own bad situation by the ravaging small-pox, and the danger of a civil war, induced the lower towns to lie dormant," Adair wrote.[61] *Variola* had indeed made its way to the easternmost town of the Cherokee Nation. In early December, a resident of Keowee, who had been among the Catawbas, died from smallpox and several others began to display symptoms of the frightful disease. Practitioners then enacted seclusion and had these infected individuals moved "some distance" from their town.[62] The arrival of South Carolina's approximately 1,700 troops on December 9 complicated such efforts to protect themselves from colonial germs.[63]

Not only did smallpox's presence make for an explosive epidemiological situation but so did the arrival of measles. This dangerous virus came to infect Lyttelton's troops along their way. Cases of the disease began to appear on November 19 and escalated over the next couple of weeks. Many men deserted.[64] At the same time, Lyttelton tried to keep his men unaware of smallpox in Keowee. He knew his militia consisted of many young colonials who likely had not gone through the infection before and might panic at the thought of the disease being so near them. After arriving at Fort Prince George, he ordered his soldiers not to cross the river and demanded that residents of Keowee burn the houses of those who had been infected and move farther away from Fort Prince George.[65] The Cherokees complied for reasons that are not stated, although they likely did not want to stay so near the encamped and measles-infested troops any more than Carolina's troops wanted to remain stationed near a smallpox-ridden Native village.

In the meantime, the governor tried to force the Cherokees to accept his terms. On December 18, Lyttelton met with Attakullakulla and five other Cherokee leaders who had affirmed that they had avoided Keowee due to the "distemper" that raged there. The indigenous leaders repeated their oft-stated view that raids on settlers were only committed by a small number of their nation, that the raids were in response to settler depredations, and that a like number had been killed on each side. Attakullakulla gave the governor a French prisoner as a gift, symbolizing his nation's friendship with the English. The following day, Lyttelton gave his answer. He would settle for nothing less than the surrender of the lead participants in the raids.[66] He blustered, "I am now come from Charles Town to this fort with a great number of my warriors, and I come prepared to take satisfaction if it is not given me." The governor added that he could do great harm to the indigenous nation, declaring, "If

I make war upon you, you will soon suffer for your rashness, your men will be destroyed & your women & children will perish for want & nakedness."[67]

Lyttelton's troops were in no shape to back up his threat. Small-pox became visibly present among them on December 27. Officers broke up the troops and moved those who had yet to have the infection to camps five to twelve miles away from Fort Prince George.[68] Given the virus's incubation period of ten to fourteen days, the initial infections of his troops could not have occurred until after they arrived at Fort Prince George. Transmission of the disease then likely occurred through clandestine communication, perhaps by way of Cherokees who went among the English in hopes to visit their imprisoned relatives or by Catawbas and Chickasaws who moved between the fort and Keowee.[69] However the disease arrived, it left the governor in a very difficult position as desertions escalated.[70] With his remaining troops riddled with disease and little time left in their three-month enlistment authorized by the assembly, Lyttelton settled for the surrender of three suspected culprits and a treaty that stipulated the release of a Cherokee hostage from Fort Prince George for each of the remaining suspects surrendered. He disbanded his troops and headed back to Charles Town on a march that was anything but heroic.[71] One British officer declared, "The Governor found himself obliged to retreat which was effected in a very disorderly manner and had much the air of a flight."[72] And to add insult to what one scholar calls "Lyttelton's folly" his troops spread smallpox throughout their colony, which suffered its worst smallpox outbreak since 1738.[73]

A very deadly situation existed back in the Cherokee Nation as well. The hostages Lyttelton took remained under British custody at Fort Prince George, and both the guards and prisoners experienced an epidemiological hell. In early January, a Cherokee hostage became ill with smallpox, prompting Coytmore to isolate him so that the soldiers would not catch the deadly disease. He could not contain the virus. By mid-January, smallpox began appearing among the British. Two died on January 18 and another the following day.[74] Coytmore became increasingly insecure and came to believe warriors from Estatoe were planning to attack Fort Prince George. Coytmore used the hostages as leverage by warning his adversaries that if they harmed his garrison, he "would put every one of [the hostages] to the sword directly."[75] Coytmore did not need his sword, at least immediately. For the next four weeks, diseases exacted a terrible toll on Cherokee hostages and their relatives who came to see them. On January 20, a Keowee woman came to the fort and soon after came down with smallpox. Coytmore had her removed to just outside the fort, where she died unattended, almost certainly sending an ominous message to those warriors who kept an ever-present lookout on the fort. The British commander had little sympathy for her as he believed she had been in on a plot in which two of the hostages managed to make their escape the day before she arrived.[76] Those two escapees almost certainly spread dreadful reports from Fort Prince George of smallpox, if not the disease itself, thus heightening Cherokee alarms of British malevolency.

The situation only got worse after the prisoners escaped. By February 4, four soldiers had died and eighteen lay "dangerous ill." Soon thereafter, several hostages took sick with what was not identified as either smallpox or measles. Among those was the Warrior of Tellico, who "died suddenly complaining of a pain in his head, loins, and back," and the "Round O" of Stecoe, who had been released from imprisonment earlier but stayed because he would not leave his captive son behind.[77] An energetic warrior for the British cause in the Ohio Valley in 1758 who came and went from smallpox-laden forts in the mid-Atlantic backcountry, Round O now suffered from war's epidemiological consequences. He finally did leave his son to the mercy of his captors and went to a Lower Town for treatment. Coytmore, rightfully worried what the consequences of the mounting deaths of the hostages would be, warning Lyttelton, "I am confident that the death of the Warrior of Tellico will enrage that town vastly and should Round O die the Middle settlement people will I imagine be for making a trial of their manhood directly."[78] Round O indeed passed on February 8, and immediately Cherokees gave "the death whoop" three times opposite of Fort Prince George.[79] Smallpox took the lives of four more Cherokees within the garrison over the next six days.[80]

As the hostages remained confined and as their deaths mounted, Cherokee warriors exacted vengeance. Several traders lost their lives during January 1760 and many others fled. War parties launched devastating raids across the frontier from Virginia to South Carolina, killed dozens of setters, captured as many more, destroyed livestock, and drove back survivors about one hundred miles.[81] On February 1, for example, warriors descended on the Long Canes settlement, killed twenty-three, and took as many captives; soon after, they descended on Stevens Creek killing another twenty-three. Settlers fought back. On February 3 they repulsed a Cherokee attack on Ninety-Six, after the warriors only gained three prisoners, including a boy, woman, and slave.[82] Several warriors lay dead and in the aftermath one colonist responded: "We have now the pleasure . . . to fatten our dogs with their carcasses, and to display their scalps, neatly ornamented on the top of our bastions."[83] Such displays did not discourage further Cherokee raids.

Cherokees even attempted a daring rescue of their confined kinsmen. Coytmore, who came to believe that warriors would not approach his outpost, reported, "As they were told by the Keowee people that we were daily burying our men and very sickly now none would continue to come near the Fort."[84] The soldiers' deaths certainly gave Cherokees some reason to think that the malevolent spirit that caused the disease, whatever its identity, did not distinguish between Natives and Europeans. Cherokees probably suspected Fort Prince George to be possessed by very dangerous spirits, if not something as deadly as Koskv Askini, then the spirits of those who had died there. Thus, it took a great deal of bravery for Oconostota or the Great Warrior of Chota to do what he did on February 16. He approached the fort and asked Coytmore for a meeting. The commander respected Oconostota's request and ventured outside of the safety of his outpost's walls. At a key moment in the discussion, the Great Warrior gave a signal and hidden warriors fired upon the exposed commander. The fort's soldiers rushed out, retrieved the dying Coytmore, and closed the gates before the warriors could rush in.[85]

What happened next guaranteed that the war would erupt with a renewed fury. The soldiers murdered all those hostages that disease had not previously executed. According to Alexander Milne, who took over for the mortally wounded Coytmore, the hostages had been in on the plot. They supposedly brandished weapons and wounded one of their guards, leading the other soldiers to open fire.[86] Whether this was the case or the soldiers simply took their anger out on their prisoners is not known. In any event, Milne claimed he did not authorize their actions and came up with an after-the-fact justification for the massacre. "Happy for us all that they were destroyed," he reported, "for searching the house where they were kept [we] found a bottle of poison, that they had hid under ground, which we imagined was to poison the well."[87] His superiors would have certainly questioned the murdering of prisoners of war since it violated European conventions, but with those prisoners supposedly plotting chemical warfare, an act that also violated those conventions, Milne supplied evidence that his soldiers need not have followed the rules. Later, James Adair commented that Milne had concocted the whole story to "excuse his baseness, and save himself from reproaches of the people."[88]

Did Milne concoct the story for an even more devious reason? Was it a cover-up for a British use of smallpox as a weapon against their Cherokee hostages? It is certainly possible but not likely. A British soldier who had previously gone through the illness could have easily transferred blankets or clothing from his comrades that lay ill with smallpox to the confined Cherokees. To date, however, no historian has seriously entertained this possibility. No infamous orders such as those that Amherst made three years later were recorded and no paid receipts for the delivery of contaminated goods have been found. Measles and possibly another disease were also present in the garrison and could not have been spread the way smallpox could have. More importantly, the British needed live hostages as bargaining chips to force their enemies to surrender those suspected of murdering settlers. The commander of Fort Prince George after all understood that should any of them die in his custody, he would be held accountable for their deaths. Ironically, Lyttelton justified his choice of bringing the hostages along with him to Fort Prince George rather than leaving them in Charles Town because of the multiple diseases that the colonial capital harbored. "Had . . . any of them died of the smallpox, or other illness [in Charles Town]," he wrote to Amherst, "it would have been believed in their nation from the jealous nature of those savages that they had been put to death of it is highly probable."[89] Lyttelton conveniently did not inform Amherst that several of those hostages had in fact died from disease in Fort Prince George and explained away Cherokee raids that escalated on British subjects during January and February as the duplicitous actions of Natives who had broken a treaty rather than what he knew to be true: he left nearly two dozen Cherokees, who had originally approached him to discuss a peace settlement, in a disease-ridden outpost where they sickened and died. This biological consequence of his hostile actions had just the result that he predicted would have happened had he left them in Charles Town. Cherokees held the British responsible for the disease-induced deaths of their kinsmen.

A new round of violence engulfed the south Atlantic backcountry in late February and March. Fierce fighting particularly occurred on the Catawba River with Cherokees taking vengeance on unsuspecting families. In doing so, they provoked brutal reprisals from settler militias. Some colonists, for example, reportedly came across a party of Cherokees in a farmhouse. The colonists set the house on fire and burnt all but one warrior to death. Dogs pursued the survivor to the river where he tried to make his escape but drowned. Settlers also repulsed a party of forty Cherokees who made an attack on Fort Dobbs. Not one warrior was said to survive, and in one of the deceased's belongings, "no less than six green white scalps" were reportedly found.[90] Cherokees nevertheless maintained the upper hand throughout the winter and spring of 1760; they brought a continual stream of scalps and prisoners into their villages and did not let up until April when raiding came to a halt.[91]

Amid the chaos in the backcountry, British colonial governments struggled to organize offensive measures. South Carolina lay prostrate with smallpox, making it impossible to mobilize its militia again and send troops back into southern Appalachia.[92] According to one doctor, *Variola* had infected some four thousand residents of Charles Town, while Lt. Gov. William Bull proclaimed smallpox as "an enemy more dreaded than Indians" for his colony.[93] The South Carolina Assembly resorted to issuing bounties to British subjects of £25 for a Cherokee man's scalp and authorizing the enslavement of Native enemies, with the proviso that men had to be sold for export to West Indies.[94] For some Carolinians, this was not enough. Patrick Calhoun of Long

Canes demanded that the scalp bounty be doubled, and the council agreed.[95] South Carolina also attempted to mobilize their remaining Indian allies—those small groups of Catawbas, Chickasaws, and Yuchis that lived in the Piedmont—by offering them rewards for scalps as well. These communities could not overwhelm the Cherokees, but they did make life more difficult.[96] South Carolina's governing council exploited their allies' dependency on trade goods. Lieutenant Governor Bull explained to the Catawbas, "As you cannot now hunt deer to clothe your women, since the Cherokee come upon your hunting grounds, you must hunt the Cherokees instead of deer, and I will take care and send clothing to King Hagler, and the women and children."[97] Governor Henry Ellis of Georgia tried to instigate an even larger intertribal conflagration by bringing the more powerful Creeks into the fray by offering their warriors £5 sterling for each Cherokee scalp taken.[98] "Nothing would contribute more to our safety than the setting those two savage nations at variance," he quipped. The South Carolina Council agreed, expressing their official opinion that "engaging the Creek Indians to go to war against the Cherokees at this juncture was a matter of the highest importance."[99] Ellis and other British officials did manage to get a relative few Creek warriors to burn the Lower Cherokee towns of Estatoe and Keowee in the spring of 1760. "I am in hopes," Ellis remarked, "that in some of these excursions the enemy will kill some Creeks whose deaths their friends must avenge."[100] Cherokees did not take the bait, however, and the two indigenous nations remained at peace with each other during the conflict.

The British also placed their hopes in smallpox. The disease had become well distributed through Keowee's population in the wake of Lyttelton's invasion. It then spread to other Lower Towns, prompting Coytmore to remark that "I can't help but being so unhuman as to wish it may spread through the whole Nation."[101] When news of the growing epidemic reached Charles Town, the *Gazette* reported with a tone of optimism "last accounts from Keowee are that the smallpox has destroyed a great many of the Indians there; that those who remained alive and had not yet had that distemper were gone into the woods, where many of them must perish as the *Catawbas* did."[102] British wishes were partly fulfilled. By February some residents of the Middle Towns began to come down with the disease.[103] When this news reached Charles Town, the *Gazette* transformed the news into a matter of fact, stating that an "abundance of Cherokees are dead of the *smallpox*."[104]

How many perished of course cannot be known but what can be known is the context in which the epidemic began. By late 1759, Cherokees understood the disease's contagious nature, had endeavored to avoid exposure, and conducted rites to close their villages off from the outside world. War inhibited their efforts to protect themselves. The disease, for example, hit the Middle Towns at the very time some Lower Town residents evacuated their settlements and retreated deeper into the mountains for fear of scalp hunters and a return of British forces. The Middle Towns, moreover, were putting themselves in a defensive posture. Warriors throughout the Cherokee Nation had been active during that winter against the British settlements, almost certainly leading to a belief that another invasion would be coming. The Middle Towns thus reduced their dispersed settlements into a fewer number of towns, "which they were busy fortifying to contain their old men, their women, and their children."[105] In such circumstances, smallpox was difficult to stop. Measles probably also spread at the time. It had arrived along with Lyttelton's troops back in December and could have caused by itself or in tandem with smallpox the "abundance" of deaths recorded in English records. In any event, Cherokee raids began to come to an end during the spring, possibly due in part to the growing health crisis in their nation.[106]

• • • •

Had the Anglo-Cherokee War ended in the spring of 1760, the smallpox epidemic may have ground to a halt as Cherokees secluded their infected kinsmen and closed off unaffected villages from contact. Colonel Montgomery's troops prevented such actions, however. On February 2 and 9, Lyttelton fired off two appeals to General Amherst to send regular forces.[107] Several days later, the governor, who was soon headed for his new post in Jamaica, escalated his pleas for assistance. He described his colony as "infested by the Indians" and called for Amherst to take "the most extreme courses" with Cherokees.[108]

As this letter made its way to Amherst and Lyttelton made his way to Jamaica, the general penned his orders to Montgomery to take charge of British efforts to punish the Cherokees.[109] On March 14 a total of 1,373 troops set sail from New York for Charles Town with orders to "act against them offensively by destroying their towns, and cutting up their settlements."[110] Unlike some three years later, Amherst made no suggestions that Britain's Native adversaries should be purposely infected with smallpox, although the general may have been aware of the germ's presence in Fort Prince George. Through Lyttelton's correspondence, Amherst received Coytmore's journal that covered the period of January 13 through 23, a period in which the disease struck both soldiers and Cherokees within the outpost. If Amherst had read the journal, perhaps it planted the seed for his future idea to use germ warfare. In any event, the general had no hesitation in ordering harsh measures against Cherokees, measures that exacerbated the impact of smallpox and made what might have been a controllable outbreak into an epidemiological nightmare.

After landing in South Carolina on April 1, British troops under Colonel Montgomery and Maj. James Grant gathered provisions, slowly made their way inland, and arrived at the Lower Towns two months later. There, they found Cherokee settlements not abandoned to the extent that they were led to believe. Residents had returned to plant crops in the spring. "The neatness of those Indian towns and their knowledge of agriculture would surprise you," one soldier stated. Another reported that Cherokee towns "abound in every comfort of life" and had "astonishing magazines of corn."[111] The invasion force made quick work of burning these towns and their food stores. The troops first sought out Estatoe and on the way stumbled onto some scattered dwellings. "Almost all the Indians in and about the houses were killed with bayonets," Montgomery reported. "A good many women and children were made prisoners, some could not be saved." The troops reached Estatoe shortly thereafter and most residents managed to escape, although some "ten or a dozen" were killed and some others tried to hide themselves in their dwellings. "Some of them who had concealed themselves were burnt in the town, which we left in ashes, and then proceeded to their other towns which all shared the same fate," the colonel further detailed. "Their loss cannot amount to less than sixty or eighty killed and about 40 prisoners, I mean men, women and children." Those who escaped left without their ammunition, clothing, and food.[112] The troops, according to Major Grant, proceeded "killing all we could find."[113]

Some Cherokees experienced an unimaginably horrific death. *Variola* still persisted among the Lower Towns, leaving some too sick to flee from the invaders. "Doubtless numbers perished in the flames, as the smallpox was in their towns, and we came upon them like lightning," one soldier exclaimed with unintended irony, not knowing that his Cherokee victims interpreted the disease from which they suffered as coming from thunder beings.[114] For his part, Amherst read news of Montgomery's actions with sadistic delight. The general congratulated Montgomery, "The success you have had . . . gives me very great pleasure as that nation will now see that we can lay waste their towns, and destroy everything they have, kill as many of them as we think proper, and show mercy to others. This indeed is the only method of treating Indians."[115]

Montgomery, though, had trouble bringing Cherokees to their knees. While some leaders advised their people to come to terms, many warriors proved unwilling. The deaths of their kinsmen in Fort Prince George, which the Cherokees made no distinctions between those from disease and violence, served as a powerful motivator to continue to resist the British. Montgomery learned: "The whole are afraid to trust us. They say they were made prisoners when they were going to Charles Town to make peace, and that some of those prisoners who were afterward detained as hostages were murdered in our fort, so that the fear of our not keeping faith with them prevents the peace being made."[116] Bull referred to the event as "the unlucky affair of the hostages" that prolonged the war and made "a peace impracticable."[117] Montgomery consequently led his troops deeper into the Cherokee Nation with the intentions of continuing the scorched-earth policy that Amherst ordered.

The colonel could not exact further punishment, however. He headed his troops deeper into the mountains, and on June 27 they ran into a considerable body of warriors just six miles before the easternmost Middle Town of Etchoe. The British were hemmed in a narrow valley and fierce hand-to-hand combat ensued. Montgomery's forces fought their way through but in doing so sustained twenty-one deaths and sixty wounded. An estimated fifty Cherokee warriors died. His troops did reach Etchoe yet found it abandoned. Residents carried off all they could, except they left a considerable quantity of corn that the British and their horses consumed or destroyed. After a few days' rest, Montgomery's forces slipped out of the town without torching it for fear that the smoke and flames would reveal their retreat. War parties continued to harass his retreating troops all the way to Fort Prince George, where they arrived on July 2.[118] At that point, Montgomery called off the offensive. He explained to Amherst that capturing Etchoe "cost us too dear" and that continuing an invasion was pointless because Cherokees would abandon their towns on approach of his forces and never trust the British enough to negotiate a peace treaty.[119] Montgomery led his troops out of southern Appalachia, arrived on the coast by August 11, presented Lt. Gov. Bull with two male and thirty-two women and children captives, and then soon thereafter departed to rejoin Amherst for Great Britain's final and successful assault on French Canada.[120]

Still, the British invasion of 1760 did considerable physical and epidemiological damage. Smallpox had simmered among the Lower Towns and made inroads into the Middle Towns in the immediate wake of Lyttelton's aborted invasion, but Montgomery's campaign enhanced the disease's spread during the summer and fall of 1760. It tagged along with the growing number of Lower Town refugees into the Middle and Valley divisions, where it raged "with great violence" according to reports printed in colonial newspapers.[121] Cherokee refugees also spread the disease to the Creeks.[122] The British received reports that the Overhills too suffered, if not from smallpox, then other diseases. Two escaped white prisoners, identified by their last names of Hosfield and Homes, found their way to Fort Prince George and reported widespread mortality. Residents of the Overhill, Valley, and Middle divisions "die very fast, of a violent disorder in their stomach and a flux," the escapees reported. A Middle Town lost sixty men, women, and children, while an Overhill Town lost thirty-five. Another Middle Town "was almost depopulated by it" and those who escaped the sickness fled into the woods.[123] Intelligence from other escaped captives contradicted the report. The *South Carolina*

Gazette reported, "By these prisoners, we do not find that the Indians have been so sickly as was represented by Hosfield and Homes and we learn that they have plenty of corn among them." Weeks later, however, Samuel Terron, an escaped trader, arrived in Charles Town and confirmed the initial report, claiming that smallpox and dysentery had in fact raged among the Cherokees in general and greatly reduced them.[124] The prospects of a terrible famine, moreover, loomed. "The crop of the Cherokee Nation of this year is not more than sufficient to support them above three months," Terron explained to South Carolina officials. "They are, particularly the Middle & Lower Settlements, almost naked, and in want of every necessary." The whole nation, the escaped trader believed, was inclined to peace.[125]

Montgomery's invasion indeed created dire biological conditions. A mass of impoverished and hungry refugees from the Lower Towns fled to other regions but found their countrymen facing a shortage of food.[126] Many Lower Town residents risked going back to their homes to harvest crops that the English had missed, but for the most part, these were short-term visits.[127] They collected what food they could and then went back to the Middle Towns.[128] There, many lived throughout the winter subsisting on "wild potatoes" after they consumed the corn that they had.[129] Many Lower Cherokees would never go back to their old towns. Instead, they built new ones, including a collection of villages along the lower Little Tennessee and Hiwassee Rivers, where non-Cherokee speakers had lived before the advent of the Native slave trade.[130] For the Cherokees as a whole, the war disrupted the ordinary subsistence cycle. Hunting suffered due to the British prohibition on trade. Cherokees obtained some ammunition and clothing through commerce with the Creeks, but it was far from what they had needed. Even if they had ample ammunition, Cherokee men could not go far to pursue game for fear of leaving their women and children behind for scalp hunters. The Overhills especially worried about going far from their villages. An army from Virginia remained camped not far from Chota and threatened to reign down destruction if the Cherokees did not surrender captives that had been taken from British settlements. The commander of these forces, Col. William Byrd III, threatened the Overhills that he would "propose soon to be in your nation; when I will not leave one Indian alive, one town standing, or one grain of corn, in all your

country, if I do not find all the white people well, when I go there."
The British, he added, were "as numerous as the fish in the sea" and
could easily drive the Cherokees into the Gulf of Mexico.[131] In response
to a feared invasion, some Overhills moved farther down the Little
Tennessee River, while women and children sought shelter to the
south in the Hiwassee Valley.[132] All Cherokees, faced a dark time of
disease, famine, and fear during the winter and spring of 1761. Before
the crops from the previous growing season ripened, many subsisted
"chiefly on acorns" and were said to be "absolutely starving."[133]

Cherokees, to be sure, tried to protect themselves from smallpox
and other diseases during the terrible ordeal of Montgomery's invasion and its aftermath. The Overhills, for example, attempted to shut
themselves off from contact. Residents of the western-most division, the English learned, were "in such dread of the infection" that
they would not allow "a single person" from the Middle Towns to
come into their towns. This same report indicated that Cherokee raids
had come to a halt and speculated among other things that Natives
ceased their warring activities to attend "their *dancing* and *physicking
days*."[134] Given the timing of this report, the unnamed ceremonies
could have been one of the regularly scheduled Green Corn festivals,
but the specter of smallpox in nearby communities may have led
Overhill medical practitioners to conduct their innovative rites to
protect against colonial germs. Whether practicing regular or ad hoc
ceremonies, Cherokees responded to the crisis that the war produced
by showing reverence to multiple spiritual beings, bringing cosmic
forces into balance, and promoting the health and safety of their
various communities. Still, it remains unclear whether the Overhills
remained safe from smallpox during the terrible year of 1760. The
flight of Lower Town refugees into the Little Tennessee Valley as previously noted served as a potential vector for diseases, if not *Variola*,
then measles or the mysterious "flux" that escaped prisoners and
traders reported as being rampant.

• • • •

Following Montgomery's retreat, Amherst's wrath against the Cherokee Nation only became worse, especially because the Overhills pulled
off something that he thought inconceivable. They captured a British

fort. Fort Loudoun remained garrisoned yet isolated on the banks of the Little Tennessee into the summer of 1760. Peace factions, most notably led by Attakullakulla, shielded the fort from a siege and in fact countenanced the actions of several women who frequently traded food to the soldiers in exchange for clothing. Angry because of the imprisonment and later murder of some of their own and emboldened by the retreat of Montgomery, warriors put an end to such friendly relations and attempted to starve the English into submission. From early June until August, the British received no food from the outside, leading many soldiers to fear starvation. On August 9, Capt. Paul Demere agreed to capitulate in return for safe passage of the remaining soldiers back to Fort Prince George. As these some two hundred soldiers walked back home, however, the Cherokees ambushed them and took the vast majority captive.[135] Amherst initially dismissed reports that Fort Loudoun had fallen but then accepted the truth after Lt. Gov. Bull confirmed what happened.[136] The commander also learned of continuing Cherokee raids, including one that resulted in the death of a Carolinian ranger and capture of a woman and two children. Amherst subsequently characterized the action as "a fresh instance of the little dependence to be made on the faith of Indians: they are, and ever will be treacherous, whenever they can commit these barbarities with impunity, no favor ought to be shown them; on the contrary they must be pursued and punished with the utmost severity."[137] He responded positively to Bull's request to send troops for another invasion that would purposely begin late enough in the growing season so that Cherokees could not plant another crop. Cherokee pacification, Amherst charged, "may be as effectively done in destroying their towns & settlements, the loss of which must of necessity make them fly to us, and reduce them to that dependence, which, and only which can secure a tranquility & lasting peace to the province."[138]

Amherst chose James Grant—now promoted to colonel—to lead the 1761 invasion of the Cherokee Nation. The general expressed his orders with even more vitriol. Cherokee actions, Amherst charged, called for "the most exemplary vengeance." He wanted Grant to use his overpowering force to "act against them offensively by destroying their towns & cutting up their settlements" and to force them to sue for "pardon & peace & the putting it out of their power of renewing hostilities." Amherst could not hide his frustration with the British failure so far to accomplish this. "I am the more strenuous in putting a speedy & effectual stop to the woes and miseries [the colonists] must undergo from so perfidious and inhuman a race of barbarians," he exclaimed.[139] Grant raised one question with his orders. "After cutting up the Indian settlements & following the Cherokees as far as troops can with any degree of safety, supposing they retire only, and don't ask for peace, what is to be done?" he asked.[140] Amherst responded: "You are to pursue the Cherokees as far as shall be practicable; to distress them to your utmost; & not to return until you have compelled them into a peace."[141] The general did not give orders to deliberately infect Britain's Native adversaries with smallpox, but he left no question that all Cherokees were to be made to suffer and to suffer severely.

Grant thus set off with his army with the intent to follow orders to starve the Cherokees into submission. His forces—totaling almost three thousand with the addition of South Carolina militiamen and some Mohawk, Chickasaw, and Catawba warriors—arrived at Fort Prince George at the end of May 1761.[142] The Cherokees faced dire conditions at the time. Reports of smallpox or other diseases had ceased, but famine stalked the land, and worries that the coming British invasion would destroy another season's harvest filled Cherokees with fear. One group of headmen sent peace overtures to the fort, claiming "they should be totally ruined, if they were prevented from planting this season."[143] They also wanted for clothing and the best source for clothes became the ransom that the English offered for their imprisoned countrymen. The commander at Fort Prince George managed to obtain the release of 113 of the soldiers who had been captured after the fall of Fort Loudon. Thirty soldiers, roughly the number of Cherokees still in the hands of the British, remained as captives.[144] Grant did take pity on some sixty starving families, allowing them to settle near Fort Prince George and make a crop, but he made his hostile intentions clear to Cherokee leaders.[145] He told Attakullakulla, "I cannot trust your people. They have broken faith so often." He further told the Overhill leader that all prisoners had to be surrendered and that continued resistance would bring his wrath:

"All those who are found in the woods & mountains will be treated as enemies. Ruin & destruction hangs over your whole Nation. . . . If any of your young men endeavor to take scalps, no mercy shall be shown."[146]

Grant's army then proceeded on its mission. They quickly burned what remained of the Lower Towns and then advanced into the Middle Towns, where again Cherokees fought back. On June 10, just before Etchoe, an estimated six hundred Cherokee warriors fired upon the advancing army for several hours, killing eleven and wounding fifty-two. Grant's scouts and rangers, however, had combed the steep slopes, killed an estimated twenty warriors, and kept the warriors too far away to inflict a more damaging blow.[147] The British commander kept his troops moving into the heart of the Cherokee Nation and gave the orders "to put every soul to death."[148] Ill supplied with guns and ammunition, the Cherokees did not offer any significant resistance and retreated. Grant subsequently had his forces burn every village they could find and "to demolish every eatable thing in the country." For a people already suffering deprivation this proved to be catastrophic. An officer in a South Carolina regiment reported, "During the whole march we found no meat in the Indian houses but horse beef; their corn mortars seemed to have had no corn beat in them for some time; they appear to have subsisted chiefly on horse flesh, and for some time past on the stalks of young corn boiled." The maturing crops that would have brought relief in about a month became subject to the British army's scorched earth tactics. "We . . . turned at least four thousand mischievous and perfidious animals to suffer miserably in the mountains," the officer retorted with dehumanizing glee.[149] Grant's men chopped down fruit trees, pulled young corn up by the roots, and burned a total of fifteen towns, two of which had been recently settled by Lower Town refugees. Altogether an estimated 1,400 acres of crops had been destroyed, an action that led the Cherokees to bestow the name "Corn Puller" upon Grant.[150]

Running out of provisions and fatigued by their activities, Grant halted his troops after a thirty-three-day rampage.[151] He returned to Fort Prince George, where he reported his results to Amherst and waited on a response from the Cherokees, believing that they "must certainly starve or come into terms."[152] Amherst commended his commander for successfully carrying out his orders. He also blamed the Cherokees for the dire biological situation in which they found themselves. In congratulating Grant, the general said, "They certainly never were so reduced and chastised but they have brought it on themselves." He also approved Grant's mercy that he showed the starving Cherokees by letting them resettle around Fort Prince George and plant their corn. Such actions would be an example of "His Majesty's lenity and protection."[153] Such leniency only came after a brutal form of warfare that had affected a wide array of Cherokees, from the very young to the oldest.

Cherokees indeed suffered extreme deprivation. A Carolinian officer reported that those Cherokees who resettled around Fort Prince George ate "old-acorns a food that we know will barely keep hogs alive." He added that "their hunger was so pinching that some of them were detected in grubbing up the grains of corn & beans after they were planted around the fort of which several officers were witnesses."[154] On top of this, these famished people had to deal with the prospect of being murdered by British-allied scalp hunters. The Chickasaws, for example, killed and scalped Ukayula or the "king" of the Middle Town of Kituwah, thus leaving a leadership void as that town's people tried to rebuild their lives.[155] Other Cherokee leaders tried to convey the extent of their people's suffering to British officers. "That the inhabitants of the towns destroyed were in the utmost distress, having scarce anything to eat, but such roots as they could pick up in the mountains, the horse flesh they used to subsist on being mostly gone," a Middle Town leader decried. "Many old people and children [were] dead and dying daily, and the young men and women that were strong and hearty, much reduced and weakened."[156] Attakullakulla informed Colonel Byrd of Virginia that "people are so starved for provision that several have been found dead in the paths & were reduced to kill their horses for subsistence."[157] Attakullakulla later informed Grant that "dying, naked, and starving" refugees from the destroyed Middle Towns had arrived among the Overhills, where provisions were already scarce. He lamented that his people had been stealing horses even from each other in order to have something to eat.[158] "I hope I shall not live to see such days again & you have destroyed our towns & our corn by which a great many of my people must die," Attakullakulla reportedly said.[159]

• • • •

After suffering terrible famine in the wake of Grant's invasion, the specter of disease returned to the Cherokees as they attempted to make peace with the British. Grant had informed the Cherokees that they needed to send a delegation to Charles Town for negotiations, but allegations of intended germ warfare complicated his plans. Grant informed Amherst that a trader named McCunningham had told Cherokees that "we wanted to kill them, that the smallpox and many other dangerous distempers were raging down the country that a great many people were dying, & that if they went to Charles Town they would never come back & that it was our intention that they should not." Most Cherokees, according to the colonel, believed every word the trader said, and if it had not been for Attakullakulla's refusal to believe what the trader said, all of the leaders would have returned home and let the war continue.[160] Grant had the trader confined, and he subsequently confessed "a great part of the story," but the colonel did "not know what to make of him" as Attakullakulla and his fellow Cherokees supplied the only evidence against him.[161] Amherst responded with his usual harshness. "I think the Indian trader who could be guilty of reporting such falsities, which might at another time prove the utmost bad consequences, ought to be punished as his behavior deserves, and should have no mercy shown him," the general exclaimed. Interestingly, Amherst expressed his contempt not at the insinuation that British officials would practice germ warfare but because a man he considered a villain threatened "to disturb the peace and quiet of a whole province, in pursuit of some private advantage of their own."[162] The general of course had no problems two years later calling for the deliberate infection of Britain's adversaries with smallpox; it was just not in his empire's interest in 1761 to have Cherokees infected during their peace negotiations.

Nevertheless, the way Amherst prosecuted the Anglo-Cherokee War had a significant epidemiological and demographic impact. The Lower Towns in general had been greatly depopulated. Many surviving residents permanently relocated to other parts of the nation and extended Cherokee settlements into the lower parts of the Little Tennessee and Hiwassee Valleys. Numbers perished during the conflict, with the majority of these casualties coming from the combined stress of smallpox, measles, other diseases, and the starvation that the British army's scorched-earth policy produced. The exact numbers of Cherokee losses cannot be known, but one British governor gave at least the perception that significant depopulation occurred. At the end of the war, Gov. Arthur Dobbs of North Carolina provided a report back to British ministers that explained that the Cherokees "were lately esteemed to be a powerful tribe, and to consist of above 3,000 fighting men, they are now upon account of the war sickness and famine supposed to be reduced to about 2,000."[163] One should of course be cautious in extrapolating a one-third population reduction of the entire Cherokee population from the governor's ballpark figures; population losses were likely not this extreme. Others shared his perception of mass mortality, however. James Adair, who remained active as a trader and led a party of Chickasaws against the Cherokees, wrote in his 1775 memoirs that other traders told him the number of warriors had declined to 2,300, when some forty years ago there had been as many as 6,000. This decline to be sure happened over a period longer than just the war, but that tragic event made Adair particularly pessimistic about the Cherokees' ultimate survival. Their losses, he claimed, were "a great diminution for so short a space of time: and if we may conjecture for futurity, from the circumstances already past, there will be few of them alive, after the like revolution of time."[164] Analyzing these same sources and others, historian Peter Wood concludes that Cherokees reached their population nadir in the 1760s, with only about 7,000 people.[165] Given the traumas of the Anglo-Cherokee, Wood's conclusion appears entirely justified.

Numbers of course do not tell the full story. Had the Cherokees been left to themselves to deal with the outbreak of infectious diseases, they likely would have fared fairly well and their population numbers would have rebounded to where they were before smallpox's arrival. Cherokees knew enough about *Variola* in 1759 to limit their exposure to the disease and cut off their villages from outside contact when an epidemic was known to be occurring. The British invasions, though, made it difficult for the Cherokees to arrest the spread of the disease. British armies gave germs the currency they needed to do their deadly damage, while their concerted effort to starve the Cherokees into submission weakened bodies for those with active infections and served as a devastating aftershock for those who had survived their bouts with colonial germs. European colonialism did not give the Cherokees much room to deal with an epidemiological crisis on their own or recover from it once it happened. The purposeful distribution of smallpox-laden blankets in other words was not necessary to punish the Cherokees to the dramatic extent that Amherst wanted.

Human agency then was very much at work in shaping the Cherokees' experience with smallpox in 1759 and 1760. Such experience, moreover, should serve as a powerful lesson in the ongoing debate about Amherst and the larger issue of intentional use of smallpox as a weapon against indigenous peoples. Scholars should be very cautious in bandying about claims that Europeans and Euro-Americans frequently used smallpox-laden blankets to advance their imperial goals. The quest to find evidence of such forms of biological warfare embarks one on a quest of futility, a futility that only adds weight to the argument that colonizers had no responsibility for the biological consequences of their actions. One might be tempted to think that without smoking guns with the fingerprints of Europeans or Euro-Americans a crime must not have been committed and colonization's depopulating impact on indigenous peoples must remain accidental.[166] Smallpox's impact on Native peoples during the British Empire's war on the Cherokee Nation, however, was no accident. British invasions created the conditions for the eruption of epidemics and undermined the ability of Natives to guard themselves against infection and mortality. Tragically, this intimate and deadly connection between germs and warfare would play out again for the Cherokees as they faced American armies during the American Revolution.

CHAPTER 4

REVOLUTION

On March 8, 1780, Cherokee warriors captured twenty-eight straggling travelers sailing down the Tennessee River and *might* have acquired
something that they surely had not wished for: smallpox. The captives, all belonging to the Stuart family, were said to be "diseased
with smallpox" at the outset of their journey. They departed from an
upper tributary of the river on December 22, 1779, and kept some
distance from the larger flotilla commanded by Col. John Donelson.
Donelson, an American militia officer, aimed to keep the disease from
spreading and even had to warn the distant Stuarts "each night when
the encampment should take place by the sound of a horn." He
seemed to have succeeded; no mention of smallpox spreading beyond
the infected family appeared in his journal, the key piece of evidence
pertaining to the voyage. Isolating the Stuarts, however, made them
vulnerable to a Cherokee attack. Many warriors from this indigenous
nation had put aside their past difficulties with the British Empire
to fight their common enemy, the Americans. Cherokees found Mr.
Stuart and his family a tempting target. Donelson recorded in his
journal, "The Indians . . . observing his helpless situation, singled
off from the rest of the fleet, intercepted him & killed & took prisoners
of the whole crew to the great grief of the whole Company." Fearing
that Natives would overtake the entire flotilla, the main group kept
moving forward despite hearing the "cries" of those left behind. The
Cherokees remained in possession of their captives while the rest of
the Donelson party completed its circuitous route down the Tennessee and then up the Cumberland to settle near present-day Nashville.[1]

What happened next to the Cherokees is not entirely clear. If anyone of the Stuarts had at the time an active case of smallpox, then the warriors may have become infected and an epidemic may have erupted. In this event, the indigenous nation shared in an experience that united peoples across the North American continent, an event that historian Elizabeth Fenn has so skillfully and eloquently reconstructed as "the Great Smallpox Epidemic of 1775–82" in her highly acclaimed book, *Pox Americana*. Fenn shows how the mobilization of navies, marching of armies, taking of captives, flight of refugees, and often poorly regulated practice of variolation spread smallpox throughout the rebellious thirteen colonies and beyond, even coming to infect Natives of the Great Plains and Pacific Northwest perhaps for their first time. This great epidemic, just as much if not more than the political struggles with the British Empire, characterized the experiences of North Americans during the years of the revolution. For Cherokees, this massive outbreak of smallpox occurred at a particularly terrible time. *Variola* made no recorded visit to them since 1760 and an entire generation of Cherokees existed in 1780 that lacked acquired immunity. Smallpox's spread thus posed a grave danger to a people trying to recover from colonialism's past traumas.

But did Cherokees actually become infected during the American Revolution? Logic seems to suggest that the Stuarts' captors must have become infected, but no hard evidence of a consequent outbreak exists. The documentary record remains silent regarding smallpox's presence in any Cherokee villages during the American Revolution. That the disease struck any Cherokees outside of their nation can only be verified with one bit of evidence: nine months after the Stuarts' capture, a British officer reported that some Cherokees then in Augusta, Georgia—two hundred miles away from the site of the attack on the Donelson party occurred—were among 140 Natives that lay ill with smallpox. The officer reported no deaths and claimed that they were "daily recovering with much nursing."[2] No other evidence demonstrates smallpox had an impact on Cherokees during the 1770s or 1780s. Pioneers, who braved the dangerous task of settling in what became the state of Tennessee, and their descendants, however, remembered something that the documents did not record: smallpox took a deadly toll on their Native adversaries. An epidemic among Cherokees became engrained in frontier folklore, incorporated into early published memoirs, and written into historical accounts of not only Tennessee's but the American Republic's founding. More recently, scholars have accepted these memories as facts and have made the Cherokees' Revolutionary War experience fit the larger narrative of colonial germs' devastating yet unintended impact on indigenous peoples.

Readers need not accept this interpretation, however. Reconsidering the Cherokees' experience with smallpox during the American Revolution should lead us into a new direction. It can illustrate how narratives that give smallpox significant credit for paving the way for Euro-American settlement are often based on problematic information, information designed to hide a darker and more troubling reality about the process in which Europeans and their descendants displaced and dispossessed indigenous peoples. Native leaders such as the Overhill leader Savanukeh knew this reality all too well, a reality in which the United States of America's independence and growth did not happen through unintended biological forces but instead by way of marauding armies that wielded nightmarish violence, weakened formerly powerful Native nations, and took lands vital for the subsistence and economic survival of indigenous peoples. Indeed, one can best characterize the Cherokees' experience during the revolution as one of total war in which multiple scorched-earth campaigns waged against them posed a far greater challenge to their survival than did smallpox.

• • • •

Reconstructing how John Donelson's journal came to be read as evidence of smallpox's supposed impact on the Cherokees in 1780 provides an interesting lesson in how historical memory becomes accepted as fact. Donelson kept a record of his party's journey in a ledger book but ceased his entries on March 7, 1780, just one day before Cherokees attacked the Stuarts. No other written document detailing what happened after March 8 existed until much later. In 1820, Judge John Haywood solicited information from participants in the Donelson voyage, and he obtained from an unknown source a poorly spelled third-person account that covered the entire time of the trip from December 22, 1779, until April 24, 1780. Haywood corrected the spelling, made some minor changes, and included the account in his 1823 book, *The Civil and Political History of Tennessee*. Meanwhile, John Donelson, Jr., who participated in the voyage that his father led, penned another version of the trip. He had kept his father's ledger, transcribed what it contained, and then filled in information regarding the remainder of the voyage. Donelson, Jr., may have written his account because of dissatisfaction with what Haywood had published, including misspelling his family's name and a few other errors, but it nonetheless closely resembled what appeared in *The Civil and Political History of Tennessee*. Donelson, Jr.'s, version ultimately came into possession of the Tennessee Historical Society, where it still remains with the label, "The Original, Journal . . . kept by John Donelson." The contents of this "original" version then became published on several occasions and was widely utilized and cited as an authentic account of events that happened during the entire course of the Donelson party's trip.[3]

Given how the "original" Donelson journal came to be produced, one should be skeptical about its contents, especially concerning the presence of smallpox. One wonders, for example, why Donelson, Sr., did not mention anything about smallpox in his ledger, but both his son and whoever informed Haywood remembered the Stuarts being infected and then inserted that supposed fact in an entry over two months into the journey. Perhaps the insertion came as an attempt to absolve the party's leader from his failure to keep those under his care from harm? In this scenario, smallpox served as a useful excuse for Donelson not keeping his party intact as it passed through the most dangerous portion of their trip. Another bit of evidence, however, seems to corroborate what participants remembered about the Stuarts' condition. On April 10, 1780, Col. William Fleming, an agent from Virginia then overseeing settlement in Kentucky, recorded in his diary that he received news that Cherokees had captured the smallpox-stricken stragglers of the Donelson party and killed thirty men, women, and children.[4] Still, the news that Fleming heard likely came from Donelson himself, who crossed paths with a surveying party that then relayed the information into Kentucky. Donelson may have immediately created smallpox as a convenient excuse for his failure to protect the Stuarts.[5]

What is most interesting, however, is not what was inserted into the journal but what was not: reference to Cherokees becoming infected. Neither Haywood nor Donelson, Jr., made any mention of the Stuarts' captors becoming sick with smallpox. Inclusion of such detail of course would have immediately made readers suspicious; the settlers would have had no way of knowing whether Cherokees became ill because they did not stick around and observe to see if smallpox's symptoms became manifest. Thus, for one to read the Donelson journal as evidence that Natives succumbed to smallpox, one would have to make an inference that the event led to successful infection.

One Tennessean who made such an inference was John Carr. In 1857, at the age of eighty-four, he became the first known person to put in writing that Cherokees suffered an epidemic in 1780. Carr recollected in his published memoirs of pioneer life in Tennessee that while he was "a small boy at the time" he heard "the reports of the great and terrible mortality which prevailed in the Cherokee Nation after the capture of Stuart's boat." He added that "Without doubt, the wretches paid dearly for their booty."[6] One must question Carr's memory, however. He was a seven-year-old resident of Virginia at the time of the Donelson party's voyage; he did not participate in the voyage but came to Tennessee some years later. There, he may have heard tales of smallpox avenging the deaths of the Stuarts, but in a letter to Lyman Draper in 1854, Carr does not refer to Natives succumbing to the disease when discussing the Donelson party.[7] His knowledge of this early attempt at white settlement in the Cumberland Valley, moreover, appears to have come directly from the published account of Haywood in 1823 and a more recent account, that of J. G. M. Ramsey, who in 1853 printed Donelson, Jr.'s, manuscript verbatim.[8] Neither Haywood nor Ramsey concluded that Cherokees in fact became infected and suffered an outbreak. It seems that between 1854 and 1857 Carr added an epidemic to his memory of events.

One can only speculate what triggered Carr to add "the great and terrible mortality" of Natives to the events of the Donelson party's voyage. But a passage he includes just below his mention of the epidemic is suggestive: "It was said that, when they were attacked with the smallpox, and the fever was upon them they took a heavy sweat in their houses for that purpose, and then leaped into the river and died by scores."[9] Carr or someone whom he relied upon for information had almost certainly read James Adair's *The History of the American Indians* and its passage on Cherokee medical personnel attempting to deal with the 1738 epidemic. Settlers on their way to Tennessee would have had no knowledge of how Natives responded to smallpox, if indeed they had a need to respond at all. The inclusion of Adair's account makes Carr's rendition appear even more fabricated. Cherokees suffered doubly—once because of punishment for their attack on Stuart's boats and then secondly because of their supposed ignorance in how to deal with a deadly disease.

Carr's memories of Cherokee mortality received greater circulation when two years later A. P. Putnam included them in his *History of Middle Tennessee*. Putnam also reprinted Donelson, Jr.'s, manuscript and cited Carr and unnamed "others" as an authority on what happened to Natives. "As the result of the capture of Stuart's boat and crew, in which were the cases of smallpox, Mr. Carr has stated, and others have affirmed the same, that 'great mortality' prevailed in the Cherokee Nation afterwards. Without doubt the wretches paid dearly for their booty."[10] Putnam also included reference to smallpox-stricken Natives leaping in the river but added one more detail about their supposed demise that reveals Adair's influence. "A large majority destroyed themselves, or died with the disease," Putnam asserted, in what is almost certainly an unattributed borrowing of the trader's claim that "a great many killed themselves."[11] Putnam went a step further and added what was at the time standard rhetoric about the demise of indigenous peoples being their own fault. The smallpox epidemic, mass suicide, "and other diseases and vices, raged among them, and so increased that the nation was hastening to extinction."[12] He concluded that in committing the murders of the Stuarts and other settlers, Cherokees invited the "judgment of heaven," which came in the form of smallpox that "destroyed hundreds of them."[13]

The Cherokees' supposed demise became written into an even more prominent narrative when Theodore Roosevelt included the anecdote in volume two of his four-volume series, *The Winning of the West*

(1889). The aspiring historian and future president narrated a version of the American past in line with prevailing Manifest Destiny ideology, wherein Providence destined an inferior race of indigenous peoples to disappear amid a tide of superior Anglo-Americans, who would spread civilization across the North American continent. The Donelson party received their due as part of this epic saga. Roosevelt used Donelson, Jr.'s, original manuscript and for the most part accurately summarized its contents. He refers to the Stuarts having smallpox, being kept at the rear of the larger group, and thus becoming vulnerable to attack. The future president, though, went off script and included the details that Carr had concocted and that Putnam later echoed. "But a dreadful retribution fell on the Indians," Roosevelt claimed, "for they were infected with the disease of their victims, and for some months virulent smallpox raged among many of the bands of Creeks and Cherokees."[14] Then Roosevelt added Adair's information for more drama: "When stricken by the disease, the savages first went into the sweat-houses, and when heated to madness, plunged into the cool streams, and so perished in multitudes."[15] While largely a summary of what Putnam had earlier published, Roosevelt added some interesting details. The epidemic raged for "some months" and the death toll involved "multitudes," a term that could easily mean that more Natives actually died than the "scores" that Carr and "hundreds" that Putnam suggested. More damaging, germs became benighted actors in Roosevelt's grand and celebratory narrative of American expansion.

Roosevelt's scholarly legacy persisted into the twentieth century. When writing the first professional historical and ethnographic account of the Cherokee people—*The Myths of the Cherokee* (1900), the anthropologist James Mooney cited Roosevelt and echoed the claim that smallpox broke out and killed "a great number" of the indigenous nation following the Stuarts' capture.[16] A later and more fully documented treatment of Cherokee history perpetuated the tale of the 1780 epidemic. John P. Brown wrote as a matter of fact that Cherokees "contracted smallpox from the captives." Brown gave no reference to his source for this statement, but he had earlier cited both Roosevelt and Putnam, from which he must have derived his estimate of "several hundred" Cherokees dying.[17] The two medical scholars

E. Wagner Stearn and Allen E. Stearn further perpetuated the story. They produced the first scholarly treatment of smallpox's impact on indigenous peoples, and they included the supposed infection of the Stuarts' captors to support their conclusion that the virus acted "as a weapon in the hands of the white man, a weapon so powerful that it was feared by the red man much more than were bullets and swords."[18]

More recent scholars have found it difficult to free their work from the legacy of the memory that a Tennessee pioneer originally created in the mid-nineteenth century.[19] Fenn, for example, includes a reference to the troubling anecdote in *Pox Americana*. Citing the Donelson journal as her only source, Fenn states as a matter of fact that while some Cherokees ventured into Georgia to help the British, "their families in the mountains of Tennessee had just picked up smallpox in an attack on some settlers."[20] She then concludes her discussion of Britain's Native allies in the South with an allusion to major population losses from disease. For the Cherokees, she states, "the pox and the war were disastrous: Having chosen the losing side, the Indians soon had to face an onslaught of Anglo-American expansion with much-depleted numbers."[21] The war part of the equation, however, remains left out of the discussion. American military actions against Cherokees are only vaguely referenced in the pages of *Pox Americana*, which in the end echoes deterministic narratives that places primacy for Native depopulation and dispossession on colonial germs rather than the colonizers' exercise of force. Fenn asserts, "*Variola* was a virus of empire. It made winners and losers, at once serving the conquerors and determining whom they would be."[22] Fenn, to be sure, does not rely on the Cherokees' supposed infection in her masterful reconstruction of smallpox's spread across North America. If Fenn had omitted reference to the incident, the larger importance of the work stands: prior to *Pox Americana*, scholars only knew bits and pieces of what was in reality a massive continental epidemic. Still, her inclusion of the problematic story of the Cherokees' supposed infection demonstrates how difficult it has been for scholars to sort out the complicated story of what really happened and what was only imagined to have happened regarding smallpox's impact on indigenous peoples.

So, must we automatically assume then that no outbreak occurred among the Cherokees during the revolution? Not necessarily. It remains possible that smallpox either by way of the Stuarts capture or through some other means made its way into the indigenous nation and spread through multiple villages. And in this event, it is possible that disease mortality went unnoticed at the time by literate British or American observers and thus remained out of the documentary record. Nevertheless, one should be careful in making too much of these possibilities. As in previous epidemics, any hypothetical outbreak during the revolution necessarily spread as a result of the marching of armies, increased volume of captive taking, flight of refugees, and other nonbiological factors. These factors also would have undermined Native abilities to defend themselves from germs, weakened the resistance of their bodies, and thus escalated mortality rates. Colonialism's violence, something the documentary record demonstrates with great detail, indeed is the paramount story of the Cherokees' Revolutionary War experience. Contemporary scholars, one can be sure, would readily acknowledge the horror that Natives faced amid brutal warfare waged against them, but the fabricated memory of a Tennessee settler that has influenced scholarly thinking should no longer be allowed to cover up the revolution's murderous legacy with a veil of smallpox.

• • • •

What made the revolution's violence especially devastating is that it occurred after a fifteen-year period in which Cherokees struggled to rebuild their communities from the upheaval of their own calamitous war with the British. The indigenous nation's leaders attempted to bring peace to their people on all fronts, sometimes in spite of British efforts to keep them at odds with other Native groups. Multiple peoples north of the Ohio bore animosity toward Cherokees. The Six Nations, especially those most closely tied to Great Britain's northern superintendent of Indian Affairs, Sir William Johnson, had helped the English against the southern indigenous nation in 1760 and 1761 and continued to send raiding parties southward in the years after. Cherokees retaliated and the cycle of violence persisted. Back and forth raids also continued between Cherokees and groups formerly allied with France, even amid the latter's struggles with the British in what became known as Pontiac's War (1763–65).[23] The cycle of violence in fact escalated during the immediate years after this event and did so with the encouragement of British officials. Johnson found it expedient to stoke the animosities between northern and southern groups to keep their attention away from settlers and to curtail the development of an even larger and more formidable pan-Native alliance from taking shape.[24] In 1766, Cherokee leaders complained bitterly about the situation. "Our enemies from the northward have attacked us this year in all parts of our country in greater numbers & more frequent than we have ever known," the Overhill Beloved Man Kittagusta exclaimed. He knew the English supplied them and asked John Stuart, the southern superintendent of Indian Affairs, to mediate a peace.[25] Attacks, though, did not abate for the remainder of the year.[26] In one raid, northern warriors killed Attakullakulla's son and seven others while they picked berries.[27] Kittagusta again appealed to Stuart to do something, claiming "we are tired of war; for our enemies were too numerous."[28] The situation became so bad that during the 1766 fall hunting season, Cherokee leaders called in their young men to protect their villages. Cherokees faced the ensuing winter with a short supply of meat for sustenance and hides for trade.[29]

To make matters worse, an epidemic of an unknown disease struck the Overhills in September and October. "When I got up this morning I could hear nothing but the cries of women and children for the loss of their relations," Kittagusta described. "In the evenings there are nothing to be seen but smoke and houses on fire, the dwellings of the deceased; I never remember to see any sickness like the present, except the smallpox." The Beloved Man begged off a request to send a delegation to join the British in marking the boundary between his nation and the colonies that they had agreed upon during the peace negotiations that ended the Anglo-Cherokee War: "If we should attempt to go to run the line, we might have been taken sick in the woods, and die, as several of our people have already been served, who attempted to escape this devil of a disorder."[30] Others confirmed that a severe epidemic had occurred but provided no details in which to make a reasonable guess as to what might have been the cause.[31] A Moravian missionary then visiting Fort Prince George, for example, only described the event as involving "great sickness & mortality."[32] What is certain is how warfare exacerbated the situation. One British officer reported, "The Cherokees seem quite dispirited in so much that they have suffered two or three straggling rascals to scalp of their people within sight of their towns without making the Least Effort to pursue them. . . . and here ends not the mischief they are afraid to go out to hunt; the trade suffers and they are starving."[33]

Amid such distress, Stuart finally gave in and agreed to pursue measures to bring about peace between Cherokees and their northern enemies.[34] It took a frustratingly long time at least as far as the Cherokees were concerned. Cherokee emissaries had traveled north in 1767 yet Sir William Johnson lagged behind in preparations for a general conference.[35] Attakullakulla and Oconostota kept up pressure on Stuart to make it clear to Johnson that they wanted "an universal peace with all the Northern Tribes."[36] Finally, in March 1768, Johnson hosted a Cherokee delegation that met with over seven hundred representatives from not only the Six Nations but a variety of Iroquoian and Algonquian groups from Canada. Soon thereafter, Cherokee diplomats traveled to Fort Pitt where they met with over one thousand representatives from the Ohio Valley and Great Lakes. Native diplomats followed up on this conference one year later with a meeting at the Shawnee town of Scioto. There, Cherokees and a variety of communities from the Great Lakes and Illinois country agreed to cease hostilities. The three conferences did not automatically end all conflict; raids and counterraids between Cherokees and northern groups occurred throughout the remainder of the 1760s.[37] But, the conferences did set the stage for a general and lasting peace among a wide variety of indigenous peoples that would have significant ramifications for the then emerging conflict between Great Britain and her American colonies.

By the early 1770s, Cherokees enjoyed a level of peace with other indigenous peoples that they had not experienced during the era of colonization. In April 1770, Oconostota thanked John Stuart for his role in bringing about the détente and expressed his delight "that our children can grow up in security."[38] Shortly before he made this statement, however, Cherokees had hosted the most important agents in bringing about this peace, Shawnee emissaries. They spread a message of pan-Native unity in the face of an expansive and aggressive Euro-American settler population that posed a threat to indigenous communities from New York to Georgia. The British worried about this emerging Native unity, especially because indigenous leaders attempted to keep their negotiations secret.[39] In one meeting at Chota, for example, Cherokees met with Shawnees, Mingos, Lenapes, and others from the north and did not allow Euro-Americans and even some bicultural offspring of Euro-American men and indigenous women to attend. John Stuart and his deputies responded by stoking animosity between Cherokees and northern Natives. They attempted to get the former to raid the latter but had no success.[40] The British interpreted what was going on through a conspiratorial lens; Natives must be plotting to attack them.[41] Cherokees, however, assured Stuart that they had no intention of warring against anyone.[42] Instead, they seemed to appreciate the decreased levels of violence and danger they faced. During the fall of 1772, for example, Cherokee leaders could send all of their able-bodied men out to pursue game.[43] "Old men, women & children walk in safety about and young men can hunt single through our nation," Cherokees told Stuart's deputy Alexander Cameron. Peace of course was not universal. Natives residing along the Wabash River still remained at odds with Cherokees. After allegedly attacking a party of Overhills and capturing six or seven women and children, Attakullakulla, despite his advanced age, led a party to avenge his people's losses.[44] Still, unlike in years past, a major flare-up of hostilities did not ensue. The Shawnees worked hard at cultivating the growing peace. In 1774, they sent a message to those communities in the north that still raided Cherokees that they should halt "shedding the blood of their red brothers and that it was time for them to unite and oppose the progress of the white people as they undoubtedly intended to extirpate [Natives] from the face of the Earth." The Great Warrior of the Overhills, Oconostota, welcomed this effort and sent emissaries to the north to foster this peace.[45]

As the rift between colonists and the British government grew, Cherokees continued to cultivate peace. In 1774, for example, hostilities between Lower Creeks and British subjects broke out. Creeks sent requests to their Native neighbors to the north for help, but Cherokee Beloved Women sent a refusal to their counterparts: "I shall take care to keep the young fellows my children at home but I see you are going to throw yours away I am for peace that my young men may hunt, while I am at home making my fire & feeding my little ones." A Lower Cherokee male leader reaffirmed the views of females: "We desire to raise our children & keep them in peace." Another Cherokee implored their neighbors to the south to listen to the Beloved Woman, "without women we could not have children."[46] Cherokees likewise gave the British the cold shoulder. Stuart and Cameron attempted to have them fall on the recalcitrant Creeks but they rejected such efforts.[47] Stuart believed that such a position was a cynical ploy due to the reversal of fortunes that the Cherokees and Creeks had experienced since the 1750s. The former suffered from the invasion of their homeland, the 1759–60 smallpox epidemic, the 1766 epidemic, and devastating losses that northern Indians had inflicted on them up until the general peace of the early 1770s, while the latter actually experienced population growth during this period. The Cherokees, Stuart claimed, "look an evil eye on their increasing numbers and superiority and wish to see them reduced to a level with themselves."[48] It is not clear whether the Cherokees wished such a fate on the Creeks; instead, they seemed to be embracing the growing view among indigenous peoples that they should stop fighting each other and focus on their own demographic recovery amid what was the most significant threat to them all, the expansion of Euro-American settlement.

Whether the Cherokees' cultivation of peace paid off in terms of demographic recovery cannot be known with certainty. John Stuart estimated that the Cherokees could field 2,800 warriors in 1764 but made no other estimate on the eve of the American Revolution to compare with his earlier estimate. Cherokees certainly had the potential to increase their population through natural reproduction, however. One of their leaders in fact revealed that his people were aware of the acute demographic disparities between his nation and the British and were consciously trying to have more babies. In 1762, the influential war leader Ostenaco had recently been in England and reported to the governor of South Carolina that he and his party found the "number of warriors and people of one color which we saw [in England] . . . far exceeded what we thought possible could be." He added that because of the recent war his nation existed in "darkness" and "distress." He thus looked forward to better days: "Our women are breeding children night and day to increase our people and I will order those who are growing up to avoid making war with the English."[49] To be sure, the continued warfare with northern Natives took a toll on his nation for the remainder of the 1760s, but after coming to peace with their multiple enemies, Cherokees could focus on having children and raising them in a relatively safe environment, a desire that their comments to the Creeks expressed. Cherokee subsistence practices, moreover, provided a key element of why one would expect to see their population grow. Corn, maize, and bean production provided a rich diet, and all indications are that cultivation of this triad flourished during the years before the revolution. In addition, Cherokees increasingly turned to domestic livestock in the 1760s and 1770s. Women began to keep hogs and chickens sometime earlier in the eighteenth century and their holdings of these animals increased in the early 1770s.[50] One would thus expect that female fertility among the Cherokees remained relatively high, at least compared to hunting and gathering tribes whose constant movement, regular periods of deprivation, and high-protein low-carbohydrate diets depressed female fertility. Such circumstances indeed support the estimates of demographic growth that historian Peter Wood has made. In 1762, Cherokee population reached as low as 7,000, while at the beginning of the American Revolution their numbers had recovered to 8,500.[51]

• • • •

Whatever their actual numbers in the mid-1770s, Cherokee recovery from violence and germs became severely threatened during the American Revolution as frictions with an expanding settler population exploded. In the years after their war with the British, Cherokees agreed to an eastern boundary that separated their nation from the colonies of South Carolina, North Carolina, and Virginia. Thousands of families rushed into areas that had yet to be settled, pushed up to the boundary, and ultimately crossed it. By 1768, colonists came to reside within a few days' walk of Cherokee towns, causing the usual

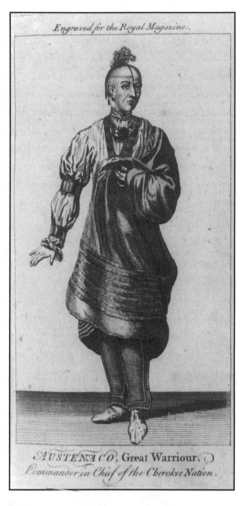

Engraved for the Royal Magazine.

AUSTENACO, Great Warriour,
Commander in Chief of the Cherokee Nation.

Austenaco [Ostenaco], *Great Warrior*, engraving by Sir Joshua Reynolds (1762). This important Cherokee leader expressed his amazement of the number of people he saw during his visit to London in 1762. He returned to find his people in deep distress yet hopeful that his nation could experience population growth. He did not foresee the tragedy that the American Revolution would bring upon his nation. (Courtesy of the Library of Congress, Prints and Photographs Division, LC-USZ62–90958)

problems that erupted when colonists and Natives came to live so close to one another: Cherokees killed strayed livestock that wandered into their territories; both sides stole horses from each other; Euro-Americans harvested game from Native hunting grounds; and members from each group ended up murdered. The historical context, however, was unusual. Settlers grew increasingly frustrated with their mother country, especially the restrictions on westward expansion, and openly defied imperial control. Indigenous peoples from New York to Georgia were caught in between. Some Native leaders struggled to keep their people out of a conflict that they believed would bring them nothing but trouble, while others saw the revolution as an opportunity to fight against the Americans in order to protect their land and resources from further expropriation.[52] Cherokees suffered severely from the violent consequences of this fight.

British officials made some attempts to stave off the growing friction between Cherokees and their Euro-American neighbors but in the end pleased no one. In the fall of 1768 John Stuart obtained Cherokee agreement to the Treaty of Hard Labor, which extended the boundary between their nation and Virginia northward to the confluence of the Great Kanawha and Ohio Rivers. The Cherokees essentially surrendered a claim to hunt in most of what is today West Virginia but maintained their claim to a vast area that includes present-day Kentucky and middle Tennessee.[53] Colonists, however, believed the area to be opened for speculation and settlement due to the 1768 Fort Stanwix Treaty with the Six Nations, who ceded it to the British based on their claim to have conquered it from other groups. Cherokees, Shawnees, and others, though, asserted that they had never been conquered and that the land remained their hunting territory. British officials agreed with Cherokee claims but proved powerless and unwilling to police the boundary. Soon after the Hard Labor Treaty, Cherokees complained that white people "pay no regard to all our talks."[54] Settlers had built farms west of the line, and Cherokee hunting grounds became inundated with Euro-American hunters and livestock. Oconostota gave the British a warning about the consequences of such violation. His young men had grown impatient and would seize all cattle and horses they found "straggling beyond the line." The Great Warrior said he would try to restrain his young men, but of the Euro-American intruders, he said, "Their daily encroachments & their killing our deer are become insufferable."[55]

In the fall of 1770, the British negotiated a new treaty designed to appease the settlers but that could not accommodate all parties involved. With the Treaty of Lochabar, Cherokees gave up more land by agreeing to demands that Virginia's boundaries be pushed farther west to the Holston River. Still, colonists defied the agreement. A large number of them took up residence beyond the border in the Watauga Valley. Older chiefs particularly Attakullakulla took pity on the Wataugans and allowed them to stay in exchange for rent, but younger warriors resented the intrusion into these valuable hunting areas. Equally disturbing, some Euro-Americans went even farther west. Under the guidance of Daniel Boone, a number of settlers ventured through the Cumberland Gap and into Kentucky in 1773.

Pan-Native opposition to this expansion enflamed the situation and increased the division between colonists and the British government. On October 9, 1773, fifteen Lenapes, two Shawnees, and two Cherokees attacked a contingent of a larger settler party and in the process killed six men, including Boone's sons James and Henry. Western settlers did not have patience for imperial efforts to deal with the situation, and one took matters into his own hands. In the spring of 1774, a wounded survivor named Isaac Crabtree killed a Cherokee man then visiting the Watuagans on a friendly mission.[56] The leader of the Watuagans, Arthur Campbell, made some effort to appease the Cherokees by informing them through Alexander Cameron that Crabtree would be punished, yet such efforts were superficial. Crabtree remained at large and eventually went to Kentucky. For his part, Campbell felt compelled to vouch for the Wataugans loyalty to Great Britain, but clearly demonstrated that such loyalty had grown thin and was conditioned on an understanding that the rights of settlers trumped those of indigenous peoples. Campbell charged Cameron and Stuart with villainous conduct by authorizing the Cherokees' use of violence and affirmed that colonists had a right to pass through the Cumberland Gap to go farther west into land that Cherokees had certainly not yet ceded. If the Cherokees resisted this movement, Campbell warned, then "a bloody & destructive war which might not end but in the total extinction of the Cherokee Nation, and the desolation of many hundreds of His Majesty's good subjects."[57]

The threat that nearby settlers posed divided the Cherokees even more deeply. Younger warriors grew even more determined to resist, while older leaders such as Attakullakulla held out hope for accommodation. Such generational tensions set the context for the infamous Treaty of Sycamore Shoals in 1775. In March, a land-speculating syndicate out of North Carolina sent Richard Henderson to negotiate with the Cherokees. Henderson asked the indigenous nation to surrender their claim to virtually all of what is today Kentucky in exchange for a vast quantity of goods. Older leaders, who especially felt the pinch of a deteriorating economic situation in which the flow of gifts had virtually ceased and debts to traders mounted, supposedly consented to what Henderson proposed. Later, these leaders denied agreeing to give up all of Kentucky, and instead insisted they ceded only a small portion of land. Because Henderson had no authorization from British authorities, John Stuart and North Carolina royal governor Josiah Martin condemned the treaty and ordered all settlers who crossed over the Treaty of Lochabar boundary to leave. Younger Cherokee warriors were most disgruntled. Their leader, Dragging Canoe, had been present at the beginning of the Sycamore Shoals meeting but left soon after it began, warning the Carolinians that he would make whatever land they settled in "dark and bloody."[58] Settlers of course ignored the orders of royal officials, whose authority over the American colonies was about to be officially severed, and risked following Boone into what would indeed become a dark and bloody land.

At nearly the same time, events at Lexington and Concord on April 19, 1775, reverberated deep into the southern backcountry. The outbreak of armed conflict forced colonists to either join the Patriots (also known as the Whigs for their opposition to monarchial authority) or the Loyalists (also known as Tories for their allegiance to the king). The former took the initiative in the South by seizing control of local governments, rooting out opposition, and in many cases driving Loyalists from their homes. Many Tories took shelter in the Cherokee Nation, where the much-hated Alexander Cameron resided. In late July and early August, Whigs from South Carolina under Col. William Thomson went to the Lower Town of Seneca on a hunt for Cameron and other Loyalists. The British agent escaped but Thomson burned the town and destroyed six thousand bushels of corn.[59] The Revolutionary War, a conflict that at least some Cherokee leaders fittingly likened to an epidemic, had come to southern Appalachia. As a Lower Cherokee speaker explained, "The great man above sent a distemper among [the Americans] which has seized the whole from Boston to Georgia, and they are now all mad. This I hope will not be our case as we intend to have nothing to say to them, for our paths to them are grown up with brush."[60]

It would be the case, however, that the "distemper"—in the form of the conflict's violence more so than in the form of actual germs—would engulf the Cherokee Nation. Late in 1775, John Stuart gave a green light to Cameron to supply Native warriors with provisions and military materials. He also sent antirebel talks to King George III's indigenous friends.[61] In April 1776, the British delivered twenty-one wagon loads of ammunition to Chota, and at the same time Cherokees came to believe that the Americans intended to send armies into the Overhills and had offered a high reward for Cameron's capture.[62] A delegation of Mohawks also visited and spread rumors that Whigs had invaded an Iroquois town and captured, tortured, and then killed Sir William Johnson's son. They also spoke of a British plan to invade from the coast while indigenous warriors attacked from the west.[63] The British indeed had such a plan and hoped Natives would act in concert with His Majesty's troops, but indigenous warriors had neither the patience nor inclination to follow imperial commands. Dragging Canoe and his warriors believed the time had come to attack their adversaries, and during the late spring and summer of 1776 his warriors joined with Mohawks, Shawnees, Lenapes, and others in a series of multipronged attacks on backcountry settlers.[64] Euro-Americans along the Watauga and Holston Rivers, who settled beyond the Treaty of Hard Labor's boundary line, bore the brunt of the attacks, although some Cherokees did cross the boundary in their attacks and did so in conjunction with over one hundred Loyalists dressed as Native warriors.[65] Most settlers escaped harm, but a general panic set in with one Virginian reporting, "The roads from Holston are crowded and numbers preparing to start on the least notice of an alarm. . . . Confusion of the people [is] beyond description."[66]

While Dragging Canoe's warriors acted without the full support of their nation, all Cherokees suffered the consequences.[67] Whig leaders believed that Native attacks were precursors for a larger British invasion by sea, and hysteria, tinged with calls for ethnic cleansing and genocide, reigned.[68] Thomas Jefferson ingrained such hysteria into the Declaration of Independence, including in the famous list of grievances against King George III the charge that he "has endeavored to bring on the inhabitants of our frontiers, the merciless Indian savages, whose known rule of warfare, is an undistinguished destruction of all ages, sexes, and conditions." To a colleague back in Virginia, Jefferson called for ethnic cleansing. "I hope that the Cherokees will be driven beyond the Mississippi & that this in future will be declared to the Indians the invariable consequences of their beginning a war," he wrote.[69] Other Americans escalated the desired punishment; one man informed his friend in Virginia, "I heartily pray that your back inhabitants may be protected from the merciless savages by the valor and spirit of its inhabitants. . . . I think no mercy out now to be shown to those devils in human shape, but to root them out man and mother's son of them."[70] South Carolina's chief justice and a member of the Continental Congress, William Henry Drayton, espoused genocide but stated he would settle for ethnic cleansing. "It is expected you make smooth work as you go," he ordered his military commanders. "That is you cut up every Indian corn field, and burn every Indian town—and that every Indian taken shall be the slave and property of the taker; that the nation be extirpated, and the lands become the property of the public. For my part, I shall never give my voice for a peace with the Cherokee Nation upon any terms than their removal beyond the mountains."[71] Griffith Rutherford, who would command North Carolinian forces, echoed such genocidal urges and called for "a final destruction of the Cherokee Nation."[72]

What followed was total war on the Cherokees. Each of the four divisions of the nation suffered the wrath of invading armies. General Andrew Williamson's South Carolinian troops converged on the Lower Towns in August 1776. One participant referred to the Cherokees as "game" but did not get much of a chance to hunt his prey, as Natives abandoned their towns on the approach of the Carolinians.[73] The same man was astonished by the bounty of Cherokee agriculture. "They were very well stored, far beyond our conception," he marveled.[74] The invaders carted off all the food they could and destroyed the rest. Every Lower Town lay in ruins, with the homes and public buildings of each put to the torch. In September, Williamson's forces converged with Rutherford's North Carolinians in the Middle Towns. The region's inhabitants fled in advance, setting the woods on fire to cover their escape, but the Americans caught up with a few stragglers. One participant recalled many years later coming upon two Cherokees, "one a squaw [who] had the top of her head cut entirely off with a tomahawk."[75] Some other Cherokees were taken alive. An officer later claimed that he at first denied permission to the men to sell the prisoners into slavery, but his men "swore bloodily that if they were not sold for slaves upon the spot, they would kill & scalp them immediately." The commander gave way on the issue and reported back to his superior that his men were "very spirited & eager for action, and is very desirous that your Honor would order them upon a second expedition."[76]

The main damage remained the scorched earth that Americans left behind. After torching the Middle division, the armies of the two Carolinas marched through the Valley Towns. There, Cherokees resisted in a two-hour battle and managed to kill or wound thirty-one of the invaders. In the end, Carolinians overwhelmed the warriors and forced them to retreat. Cherokees left supplies that they would need to survive the upcoming winter, including a large quantity of "blankets, moccasins, boots, some guns, matchcoats, deerskins, &c, &c." After this brief fight, the total war continued. One soldier reported that at the first Valley settlement the troops "spread through the town to destroy, cut down and burned all the vegetables belonging to our heathen enemies, which was no small undertaking, they being so plentiful supplied." Cherokees had a vast number of hogs as well as "great apple trees, and, whiteman-like improvements." These were quickly destroyed. Most Cherokees again managed to escape before the troops arrived, but North Carolina's soldiers managed to surround one town before all of its inhabitants vacated and killed an unreported number of them.[77] Americans surprised another group and captured sixteen individuals, largely consisting of Tory traders and their wives and bicultural children. Most of these would later return to the Cherokee Nation, but an untold number of others were not so lucky. One soldier, for example, captured a lame woman and immediately killed her, while another soldier killed an elderly prisoner that he had in his possession.[78]

Meanwhile, Virginia's forces bore down on the Overhills. On October 18, Col. William Christian and his forces of over one thousand men arrived on the Little Tennessee. He met with no opposition as he went through the first four towns along his route: "The Indians had ran off hastily. . . . Some of them had shut their doors and some had not: they had carried off their clothes & best of their household goods but took but little provisions, the greatest part of them I judged went off in canoes down the Tennessee."[79] The colonel found abandoned livestock and fields that he estimated would yield "between forty and fifty thousand bushels of corn and ten or fifteen thousand bushels of potatoes." Unlike the Carolinians, the Virginians paused before commencing any destruction. They treated with relative kindness "an old woman and two children" by giving them food after they had been in the woods for six days and nights.[80] They also took in "a young man who had lost his wife and was then in search of her." The man told the Virginians that his people "were so much afraid that they would fly before us wherever we went."[81] The Overhills had certainly learned the fate of their nation's other divisions and feared they would end up enslaved or killed if they remained.

Christian made some effort to distinguish between hostiles and those who would agree to peace. The colonel suggested to Gov. Patrick Henry that such an effort would be a more honorable course for their state: "I know six [Cherokee leaders] that I could kill & take hundreds of them, and starve hundreds by destroying their corn, but it would be mostly the women and children as the men could retreat faster than I can follow and I am convinced that the Virginia state would be better pleased to hear that I showed pity to the distressed and spared the suppliants; rather than I should commit one act of barbarity in the destroying a whole nation of enemies."[82] Perhaps the Carolinians prior efforts weighed a bit on the colonel's conscience? Christian sent a request to Savanukeh to discuss terms, which above all else meant the surrender of Cameron, whom settlers held most responsible for instigating indigenous violence. The Virginians, though, did not receive what they wanted and took punitive actions. Joined by three hundred North Carolinians, Christian's forces spared Chota and some other towns but destroyed the five towns perceived to be most hostile.[83] The punishment was as severe as what towns in the nation's other divisions faced. Joseph Williams, one of Christian's officers, later recalled that the Overhills "had great numbers of fat cattle and hogs, with poultry of every kind in abundance." The soldiers consumed or drove off the livestock and either burned or destroyed the Natives' "immense quantities" of corn.[84] Without their harvest, livestock, shelter, clothing, and bedding, many Overhills faced the ensuing winter of 1776–77 as starving and exposed refugees.[85]

• • • •

Well before they had supposedly succumbed to smallpox, Cherokees had suffered severely from the Revolutionary War's violence. To make matters worse, there appeared to be no end in sight to the brutal conflict. Some Cherokee and Whig leaders certainly wanted to end the strife and negotiated a settlement of sorts. It included the punitive Treaty of DeWitt's Corner (May 1777) and the Treaty of Long Island of the Holston (July 1777), which together required Cherokees to surrender substantial quantities of land.[86] This settlement, however, only added strength to Dragging Canoe and his faction. They rejected the land cessions, withdrew from the larger nation, moved south to the bend of the Tennessee River, and established several towns on Chickamauga Creek, from whence they received their name.[87] The Chickamaugas continued to receive supplies from the British and raid Americans.[88] Many Lower Cherokees also remained violently opposed to accommodating the Americans and moved farther to the west into the upper Chattahoochee and into the many tributaries of the Coosa in what is today north and northwestern Georgia.

Whig settlers, moreover, did not abide by the treaties and provoked otherwise peaceful men to either support or join the militant towns. Cherokee leaders who hoped for a cessation of conflict were put in a difficult position. In April 1778, for example, Savanukeh, who by this time emerged as a powerful speaker for the Overhills in the wake of Attakullakulla's death from old age and in the wake of Oconostota's departure for the Chickamaugas, warned the Americans about the consequences of further encroachment: "My people have been lying very still. They had good ears at the treaty, I wonder at your people of Watauga, that they should be so forgetful, they are marking trees all over my country, and near to the place I live, and are killing my stock near my beloved towns." He then complained about the Whigs' failure to punish such trespassers.[89]

As 1779 began, a British invasion of the South reinvigorated Cherokee opposition to the Americans. On December 28, 1778, over three thousand British, Hessians, and Loyalists retook Savannah, Georgia.

This invasion began the British high command's southern strategy. Failing to subdue the rebels in the North, the British would send the bulk of their military personnel to the South, a region mistakenly believed to have a Loyalist majority who could join with regular troops to destroy the Whigs. The British believed Natives—particularly the Creeks and Cherokees—could be of great assistance in this strategy.[90] In January and February, John Stuart from his headquarters in Pensacola sent intelligence of the plan to Britain's indigenous allies and gave promises of increased supply of munitions.[91] Chickamaugas and Lower Cherokees greeted such turn of events favorably as did a growing number of warriors who remained in the old towns and had previously come to terms with the Americans. The Cowee Warrior, for example, claimed that he had "been long waiting for" news that the king's troops had arrived and would consequently set off to war. "The Rebels drove me from my land," he explained, and now "I have got help [and] hope to drive them from it." At the same time, the Cowee Warrior worried that "my people are apprehensive of the rebels taking the advantage of our absence & destroy the women & children but I hope the King's troops will keep them busy at home."[92]

The Cowee Warrior's worries were well placed. As Cherokee men ventured into Georgia to help the British, Whig forces attacked. Governor Thomas Jefferson of Virginia, receiving information of escalating raids on western settlers, ordered Col. Evan Shelby to lead some nine hundred North Carolinians and Virginians on a punitive expedition against the Chickamaugas. In April, they sailed down the Tennessee, surprised the Chickamaugas' five towns, destroyed each, burned some twenty thousand bushels of corn, killed or herded away all the horses and cattle that could be found, confiscated goods valued at £25,000, and delivered "a very threatening Talk" to a Native woman who was to relay it to the absent warriors.[93] How many deaths the Chickamaugas sustained is unclear. Jefferson reported that his forces killed "a dozen" but did not specify the age or gender of those killed, while Cameron in one letter claimed that the Americans killed two men and two women and in a later letter claimed that a total of five women and children had been put to death.[94] In any event, the invasion had mixed strategic results. Coming in April, it did not undermine Cherokee subsistence as had previous invasions. Chickamaugas rebuilt towns, although perhaps in new locations, and were able to plant crops for the 1779 growing season and continued both to aid British forces and raid American settlers.[95] Cameron reported, "They keep continually killing & scalping in Virginia, South Carolina & the frontiers of Georgia although the rebels are daily threatening to send in armies from all quarters & extirpate the whole tribe."[96] Still, the defeat led to turmoil among Cherokee militants. Oconostota proclaimed his readiness for peace. "It was bad white men that were always setting us on to war but now we are determined to do so no more," he told Shelby. He added that he intended to move back to the Overhills after the fall harvest.[97] Many younger warriors, though, remained vehemently opposed to accommodating the Americans and continued the fight.[98] The Chickamaugas remained a potent fighting force and would increasingly attract individuals of diverse backgrounds including a large number of Euro-American Loyalists and Creeks.

At the time of Shelby's campaign, *Variola* had just begun to make inroads into the South and approached the Cherokee Nation from many directions. In April, American forces under Gen. Casimir Pulaski marched from the north to counter the British invasion but brought the virus with them and infected a community of Moravian settlers in Salem, North Carolina.[99] Cherokees had learned of the approaching disease and acted with caution. In May, a delegation of the "peaceable towns of the Cherokees" set out for Williamsburg to negotiate with Governor Jefferson, but their leader, the Hanging Maw, turned his party back home after "hearing that infectious disorders such as the smallpox &c are raging in the lower parts of Virginia."[100] Smallpox approached the Cherokees from the south as well. In February, British ships arrived at Pensacola with infected soldiers. Officers tried to enact quarantine but desertions of the sickened troops escalated.[101] By June, "numbers" of British soldiers and Loyalist refugees were reported as dying every day from smallpox and other diseases.[102] Somehow *Variola* made its way into Creek towns, perhaps by way of the deserters that fled Pensacola or by way of Creek visits to the British outpost. By fall the disease had taken a significant toll on the Creeks. Cameron reported from their nation that they "seem to be tired of war . . . besides the smallpox has reduced them much, and those towns who have not had it as yet, have fled with their families into the woods."[103] Word of the outbreak found its way into the American press. The *Pennsylvania Gazette* reported that smallpox raged "most violently among the Creek Indians at present, so that they will hardly be able to do anything for their British brothers this campaign."[104] Americans probably wished for the same to happen to the Cherokees but such wishes appear not to have been fulfilled. Alexander Cameron resided among the Cherokees from June 28 until September 27, and in his 1779 correspondence he made no mention of smallpox among them.[105]

What more certainly plagued Cherokees was another American invasion. In August, General Williamson led his South Carolina militia against the Lower Cherokees. Cameron had been residing among this division, and Whigs wanted nothing more than to capture the hated British agent. He eluded their grasp, however, and Carolinians did what they did best: they burned six to eight towns, destroyed fifty thousand bushels of corn, and killed or herded off whatever livestock they could find.[106] Williamson gave no official count of the number of Cherokee deaths but one of his soldiers later recalled killing "a considerable number."[107] While the number put to the sword cannot be known, all residents suffered extreme privation as a consequence of Williamson's scorched-earth tactics. Cameron reported that as result of the lost harvest, the Lower Cherokees were "living upon nuts & whatever they can get." He purchased 300 bushels of corn to feed Britain's starving allies, but it was 49,700 bushels short of what they had before the South Carolinians invaded.[108] He added that Williamson had "reduced and distressed them to the utmost misery."[109] Once again made refugees, Lower Cherokees fled their destroyed villages and relocated to what they hoped would be the more difficult to find locations in northwestern Georgia.[110]

It was within one year of Williamson's and Shelby's campaigns that the great smallpox epidemic of the revolution supposedly began its leg through the Cherokee Nation. But, again no evidence dated to 1780 confirms this. The Chickamauga's capture of the Stuarts in March of that year, to be sure, may have led to infection, if the captives had active cases at the time of capture and if the captors lacked acquired immunity. In this event, if practitioners did not act quickly enough to seclude those beginning to show symptoms, then the virus could have become dispersed through multiple villages. Nevertheless, one should not automatically jump to the conclusion that a successful transmission occurred or exaggerate the possible impact that this supposed transmission had. It may be the case that Cherokee warriors who were exposed to the disease were not susceptible. Some of them may have acquired immunity by surviving infections contracted during the smallpox epidemic of 1759–60. Younger warriors in their teens of course would have been vulnerable, but transmission was not certain simply because Natives were involved. The Stuarts, moreover, may not have been as viable of a vector as they first appear to be. Recall that the Donelson party began its journey on December 22, and the Chickamaugas captured them on March 8. Did the Stuarts maintain a chain of infection over this more than two month period? By the time of the incident, smallpox may have run its course through them, unbeknownst to Donelson, who had limited contact with the stragglers as he kept them away from the larger group. Lastly, supposing transmission occurred from an infected captive to a susceptible Chickamauga warrior, one should not assume the disease inevitably spread. To assume so, would be to deny what more in-depth research clearly shows: practitioners could have quarantined infected patients, closed off unexposed villages from outside contact, and thus stifled *Variola* before it ignited a more widespread epidemic.

Protecting themselves from smallpox in fact figured prominently in Cherokee decisions relating to their participation in the larger British campaign of 1780. In that year the British sent more troops into the southern theater with the aim of capturing Charles Town. They hoped to have Native assistance in doing so, but smallpox complicated the plans. Due in part to variolation, the disease had proliferated in Georgia during the first few months of 1780.[111] At the same time Col. Thomas Brown invited indigenous warriors to meet with him in Savannah to receive gifts, supplies, and intelligence about British plans. He had taken over as British superintendent of Cherokee and Creek affairs after John Stuart passed away the previous year and after Alexander Cameron received a transfer to work among the Choctaws and Chickasaws. Over three hundred Cherokees whose villages had been destroyed by Williamson made the trip and arrived in Savannah in early March.[112] With smallpox present there, Cherokees did not want to stay long.[113] Brown reported, "Having held a conference with the Indian chiefs on this subject, they told me, they were willing & ready to give every assistance in their power to the Great King & . . . but that as the small pox . . . raged throughout the province, they would not be able to prevail on their young men & warriors to remain under their present apprehensions of receiving an infection." Cherokee leaders supported their apprehensions with a reference to "a former occasion" in which they "sustained a loss of 2500 men," likely due to the 1738–39 epidemic that they may have survived during their younger years or that they learned about from their elders. In any event, they fully knew the dangers of the disease and warned the British "if only one of the party was infected the others would disperse & run into the woods." Brown concluded "that it would be highly impolitic in the present juncture to hazard our Indian interest by exposing them to a contagion so fatal."[114] The Native warriors consequently went away to "shun the smallpox."[115]

The escalation of Cherokee military activities at the end of 1780 suggests that Cherokees put up a successful fight against smallpox, and the disease had very little impact, if any at all, on their nation. Again, the only direct reference to any members of the indigenous nation becoming ill with the disease comes from the pen of Colonel Brown, who reported a mild outbreak in December among a relatively few who remained garrisoned with the British at Augusta. In the same letter, Brown bragged about his successful encouragement of the Cherokees to attack the Americans. Britain's Native allies, the colonel reported, were striking the "plunderers and banditti who have taken forcible possession of their hunting grounds" in not only the Watauga and Holston Valleys but also those farther west along the Cumberland where the Donelson party had recently arrived. Cherokee raiders also hit newly established Kentucky settlements and would-be settlers who ventured down the Ohio.[116] Such actions, moreover, had a tangible impact on the course of the larger Revolutionary War. In October, Britain's southern strategy suffered a devastating blow when Whig militias from the backcountry routed Loyalist forces at King's Mountain in western South Carolina. With his troops exposed to an assault from the west, Cornwallis retreated to the coast for the winter, but he did so without harassment. Whig militias from the backcountry turned back after learning of Cherokee attacks. Corn-wallis's increasingly undermanned and ill-supplied army lived to fight another day.[117] Had Cherokees been suffering from a major outbreak of smallpox in 1780 it is doubtful that their military activities would have had such an impact.

• • • •

American militias rather than smallpox proved to be the deadliest scourge that threatened the Cherokees. Whigs sought to inflict severe retaliation against Natives who had accepted British talks urging them to escalate their raids.[118] In late December 1780 and early January 1781, John Sevier led 250 soldiers into the Cherokee Nation and defeated a large body of warriors on the way. Arthur Campbell's force of 400 joined Sevier's troops and together proceeded to the Over-hill and Valley divisions. At one point, the Beloved Woman Nanyehi approached the Americans and "made an overture in behalf of some of the chiefs for peace." Campbell reported that he "evaded giving an explicit answer, as I wished first to visit the vindictive part of the nation." Campbell got his wish. The Americans attacked ten towns including Chota, burned one thousand homes, and destroyed fifty thousand bushels of corn. He reported killing twenty-nine Cherokee men and taking seventeen prisoners, "mostly women and children." At one point, the soldiers "drove several into the river," where they likely drowned or died of hypothermia. Americans only lost one man.[119] Before leaving, Campbell and Sevier gave the Cherokees a threatening message. They chastised warriors for "listening to the bad councils of the King of England, and the falsehoods told you by his Agents," encouraged them to drop out of the war, and called for them to accept a defeat that left Americans in possession of the contested lands.[120]

Many Cherokees were unwilling to accept this. Even as Campbell and Sevier razed Overhill and Valley Towns, Cherokees conducted raids into American settlements and would continue to do so during the early months of 1781.[121] Campbell appealed to Jefferson to autho-rize further retribution. This time Campbell wanted the Lower and Middle Towns "desolated" as "the want of Bread would cause many

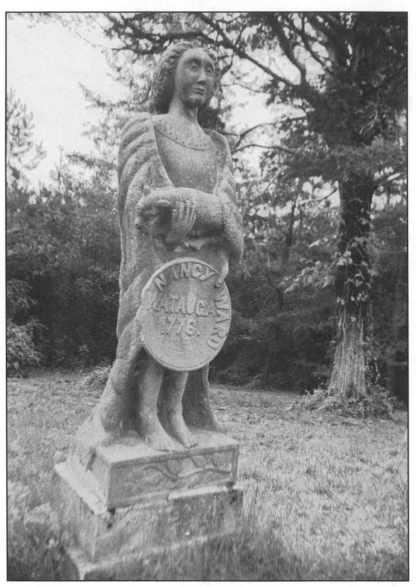

Nancy Ward, statue by James Abraham Walker (ca. 1912), photograph by Ray Smith, August 1975, http://smithdray.tripod.com/nancyward-index-5.html. Cherokee women expressed their ardent hopes to maintain peaceful relations with all people during the early 1770s so that they could rebuild their depleted population. Among those was Nanyehi (known to Euro-Americans as Nancy Ward). During the winter invasion of 1780–81, John Sevier ignored her appeals to spare Cherokee villages. To add insult to historical injury, the statue of Nancy Ward was reportedly stolen in 1980, made its round on the commercial art market, and has yet to be returned to its home in Arnwine Cemetery near Liberty Hill, Tennessee. (Photograph used with permission of Ray Smith)

other wants, which would soon lower their vindictive spirit." Sevier returned to do just that, although managing just to strike the Middle Towns. Reports of the damage he inflicted vary. Campbell claimed Sevier "destroyed three principal towns with some scattering villages, killed upwards of twenty Indians, and brought off fifteen prisoners, mostly children."[122] Another Virginia official claimed Sevier destroyed six towns in all, killed thirty, took nine prisoners, and absconded with two-hundred horses.[123] The Cherokees perhaps best captured what really happened. One delegation that approached the Americans in April about peace reported that their people were then "perishing in the woods & eating roots."[124] Savanukeh later decried that as a result of the American invasions in December and March "our families were almost destroyed by famine" during the ensuing spring. The Cherokee leader would remain opposed to the Americans until the end of the war and would harbor resentment toward a people that he claimed had "dyed their hands in the blood" of his people.[125] Colonel Brown who received Savanukeh's talk added his own comment that "the wanton bloody outrages therein mentioned, committed by the rebels on such unfortunate Indian women and children as have fallen in the course of the war into their hands, have been truly barbarous and more than savage."[126]

More was yet to come. Throughout 1781, Whig forces steadily regained control over the southern backcountry, including Augusta, which fell to the Americans in June. Many Loyalists fled into the Cherokee Nation and joined with Native warriors on raids against Whig settlements.[127] Retaliation came with swift brutality. In November, Gen. Andrew Pickens of South Carolina and Col. Elijah Clarke of Georgia combined forces on an eleven-day campaign against the Lower Cherokees. Clarke left the only first-hand written account of what happened, reporting "with pleasure" that the mounted Whig militiamen killed "about" forty Native men and two Loyalists, burned seven towns, and destroyed "some thousand bushels of corn and a large quantity of other provisions." Clarke also added that the soldiers pursued those who tried to escape, found and killed some of these, and discovered and then destroyed "some hundred" bushels of hidden corn.[128] Later recollections by a participant painted an even more vicious picture. Whig militiamen relied on swords because of a lack of ammunition and were supposedly told "to kill all who had the appearance of warriors." As the sun rose and their "swords glittered in the rays," they surprised the town of Little Chota on the headwaters of the Chattahoochee. The frightened residents fled in every direction as the attack began, while the troops "broke & pursued generally in squads cutting down the Indians with their swords—if one blow failed of the object, a second or a third from some of the others, did the work." One soldier, described as "a very large & powerful man," used his large sword to "cleft upon the heads of the flying Indians like so many pumpkins." Another soldier chased a Native into a ravine, decapitated him, and then stabbed the head repeatedly. This same account puts the loss of life much higher than what Clarke reported. Seventy-nine Cherokees reportedly lost their lives, while "about forty aged Indians, women & children" became prisoners during the "bloody day's work."[129] The exact number of dead will never be known but whatever it was it certainly included some Cherokees who perished during the following winter months from cold, exposure, and starvation. Later, Colonel Brown offered a grim picture of how the Cherokees suffered: "Numbers of their women and children have been butchered in cold blood or burned alive, yet no species of rebel barbarity or the loss of their towns, provisions, families or friends have induced them to abandon His Majesty's service."[130]

Many Cherokees in fact remained committed to fighting—not on behalf of King George III but to protect their own lives and lands— even after Cornwallis's October 19, 1781, surrender at Yorktown.[131] Along with remnants of Loyalist militias, Native warriors kept the southern backcountry in a state of war. In late November, one of these combined groups in fact captured a wagon train hauling munitions to Whig forces, apprehended Andrew Pickens's brother John, and reportedly turned him over to the Cherokees, who supposedly tortured and killed him.[132] Pickens of course was angry about the death of his brother, whoever killed him, but on top of this, the situation in the Long Canes and other western settlements had grown dire. Years of war had disrupted planting and scattered their livestock, and with the general economy in shambles, some settlers got a taste of what the Cherokees were all too familiar with: they had to eat roots, wild fruits, and whatever else they could scrounge from the woods.[133]

Pickens in fact worried that "unless some spirited measures are taken and immediately carried into execution against the Cherokees and Tories that are harbored in the nation—this part of the country must be evacuated for some time."[134] The Whig general wanted more than to round up militant Loyalists and warriors; he saw the Cherokee Nation as a potential source of food for hungry settlers.

In March 1782, Pickens's forces scavenged what they could from the Cherokees. He had originally proposed a joint operation with North Carolinian forces, one in which his army would proceed through the Lower Towns to the Chickamaugas, while the latter would come down from the north into the Middle Towns. The two forces would then converge in the Valley Towns.[135] The plan did not proceed as Pickens hoped. Cherokees discovered his approach and abandoned their towns in advance of his forces. Pickens in fact never made it to the Chickamaugas and became disappointed that his intended targets in the Valley and Lower Towns took all of the food with them as they departed for their hiding places in the mountains. He complained about finding only forty bushels of corn and "four small beeves" in all.[136] Meanwhile, North Carolina's forces under Joseph McDowell got off to a late start and never joined with Pickens. They scoured the Middle Towns for about two weeks and managed to take some prisoners before turning back home.[137]

While not having the results that Pickens wanted, the return of Whig forces in the winter served as a damaging aftershock to the previous fall's invasion and brought more turmoil for all Cherokees, whether neutral or actively engaged against the Americans. Evan Shelby described the Cherokees during the spring of 1781 as "in a deplorable situation being naked and defenseless for want of goods and ammunition." He learned that men from friendly towns would not venture out to pursue game for fear of being mistaken for militant warriors and killed, which had recently happened to some Valley Town hunters. Shelby wrote, "I cannot help pitying the wretches and have promised them we would use our endeavors for to have them furnished with the most needed necessaries."[138] American officers, however, were in no position to help. They lacked the resources to offer material aid, and they could not control the settler population that caused such strife. During the summer of 1782, another round of Native raids occurred. Lower Cherokee and Loyalist war parties again swept the Long Canes, while Chickamaugas led attacks against American settlements in the upper reaches of the Tennessee watershed.[139]

In response, Whig governors of the southern states authorized the largest strike against the Cherokees since the 1776 combined invasions. Scorched-earth tactics were again to be used. Pickens took the lead in calling for the punitive actions. The Cherokees, he claimed, were a "people who only can be brought to measures by fear or necessity, & as they can have the mountains for shelter, & their corn can be had there for their support, I fear it will be difficult to reduce them to measures, but we must do what rests in our power, to disconcert their plans."[140] Pickens's forces set out for the Lower Cherokees in late September and centered their actions on the recently relocated villages on the Etowah River. The only surviving report he made immediately after his campaign provided few details about what happened, merely stating that "a considerable number of [Indians] were made prisoners" and that he forced the Cherokees to agree to peace and surrender to him any Loyalists that they had among them.[141] Participants later recorded in their recollections destroying several towns and killing "several Indians" but do not give many details either.[142]

Perhaps they had something to hide. That is exactly what the commentary of Col. Thomas Brown suggests. Writing in 1786 in response to a Whig historian's condemnation of him employing "savages" during the revolution, Brown accused the Americans of acting more brutally than Britain's Native allies ever did. He particularly lambasted Pickens for producing "a scene of devastation and horror!" "Thirteen villages destroyed," Brown exclaimed. "Men, women, and children thrown into the flames, impaled alive, or butchered in cold blood! How different the conduct of those you style savages!"[143] Pickens may or may not have been made aware of Brown's condemnation, but he seemed concerned about how his actions against the Cherokees might tarnish his reputation. After the revolution, he had become a leading man in state and national politics and during a term in South Carolina's House of Representatives he narrated his war experience. He put the onus of brutality back on the British by referring to Colonel Grant's 1761 invasion, an event that he participated in as a young man. "Then I learned something of British cruelty which I always abhorred."

He added that during his Revolutionary War campaigns against Natives "I issued positive orders that no Indian woman, child, or old man or any unfit to bear arms, should be put to death on pain of death on the perpetrator giving at the same time the object I hoped to obtain by it." He claimed that his men obeyed his orders and set an example that Natives themselves followed.[144] Even if Pickens is to be believed, however, his actions had a devastating effect on Natives of all age groups and sexes that cannot be hidden by selective memories. His scorched-earth invasion left numbers of Cherokees to face another winter as homeless, hungry, and exposed refugees.

So too did the actions of John Sevier and his troops who struck other Cherokee towns at the same time.[145] Sevier passed by the already pacified Overhills and instead concentrated his troops' activities against towns along the lower Hiwassee River, Chickamauga Creek, and the Coosawattee and Oostanaula branches of the Coosa. "We destroyed all their towns, stock, corn, & everything they had to support on," Sevier's son James, who participated in the campaign, later recalled. He added that the "Indians eluded our march and kept out of our way in the general, although a few men, women & children were surprised & taken." These prisoners the younger Sevier claimed were all exchanged for captive Americans on the army's return march through Chota. Not a single American was reportedly killed in the campaign, while the number of Cherokee casualties remains uncertain. James Sevier did not indicate that the Americans killed any Natives, but other veterans gave vague impressions that they did.[146] One participant recollected "burning and destroying wigwams killing and taking the natives prisoners," while others stated that they had "killed a number of Indians," "killed several," "killed some 18 or 20 Indian warriors," and "killed some of their men."[147] Whatever the casualties, Sevier inflicted a major defeat on his adversaries. Cherokees abandoned Chickamauga Creek and moved farther down the Tennessee, where they established the five new towns of Lookout Mountain, Crow Town, Long Island Town, Nickajack, and Running Water. Other refugees returned to the Cherokees old towns and did so in a desperate condition. Colonel William Christian predicted "hundreds" of Cherokees would die of starvation. They were "almost naked," he claimed, and "their corn and Potatoes, it is supposed will be all done before April. And many are already out, particularly widows and fatherless children."[148]

It was just amid such dire conditions that one would expect that infection and mortality—if it was indeed a problem for Cherokees—would have been most severe. Neither British nor Americans at the time, though, made any such reference to an epidemic. Neither did the Cherokees themselves. In January 1783 Cherokee leaders appealed to Col. Brown to not forsake them, especially considering all that they had endured. They traveled to Saint Augustine, where Brown and other British officers had relocated, and described their distress. The main speaker of the group recited: "I received the talk of the Great King and raised the hatchet and have lost in different engagements six hundred warriors, my towns have been thrice destroyed and my cornfields laid waste by the enemy. As a man I performed my word. . . . I hope therefore [the British] will not forget the talks themselves and abandon their friends to the resentment of their enemies."[149] But that was just what the British did. With the Treaty of Paris in 1783, the Revolutionary War between Great Britain and the Americans came to a formal end, leaving Cherokees and countless other indigenous peoples to face the aggressively expanding new republic of the United States of America largely on their own.

• • • •

Even without a smallpox epidemic, the American Revolution proved to be an utter catastrophe for Cherokees. As in the other episodes in their history, colonialism escalated violence and created traumatic living conditions in which they found it difficult to recover from population losses. The Americans' scorched-earth tactics caused immeasurable harm and led to numerous deaths from starvation and exposure. The trauma would continue beyond 1783 as Euro-American settlers flooded west, the Chickamaugas continued to resist, and American militias retaliated with the same scorched-earth tactics used during the revolution.[150] A general peace was not achieved until 1795, and when it came, it did so at the cost of millions of acres of land that Cherokees had to cede to the United States. Such violence stifled the Cherokees' brief period of recovery between their war with Great

Britain in 1759–61 and the revolution. Historian Peter Wood posits that Cherokee population fell to 7,500 in 1790—only 300 above his estimate for its nadir after the Anglo-Cherokee War.[151] Smallpox did infect at least a small number of Cherokees confined with the British at Augusta and may have been more widespread, but the Americans did not need to introduce the deadly disease, either wittingly or unwittingly, to produce a dire health crisis for Natives they sought to conquer. By waging a scorched-earth policy, something completely intended, they purposely altered material conditions knowing that severe human suffering and fatalities would result.

The memory of frontier settlers—first put in writing by John Carr in 1857—hides this intended trauma. The writing of this memory into historical narratives as fact exemplifies something deeply problematic in the larger literature on the European introduction of novel germs. This literature has come under increasing scrutiny and criticism, and to this critique one can add that many historians have been misled by unsubstantiated claims that have found their way into their analyses.[152] Perhaps it may be as historian David Jones states that the use of "morally neutral bio-historical forces" has great interpretive appeal and leads both academics and a lay audience to accept with little question the "virgin soil" thesis and otherwise determinative interpretations of history as those offered by Diamond and Mann. As this chapter shows, however, narratives of disease are anything but morally neutral.[153] Non-Natives told stories of smallpox's impact on their indigenous adversaries for a reason, and scholars have utilized these stories complacently and uncritically. Narratives of disease thus continue to be told that obscure how colonialism—in all its manifold yet connected aspects—has negatively impacted indigenous health and well-being.

CHAPTER 5

VACCINE

Till forth their chiefs o'er dying thousands trod
To seek the white man and his bounteous God:
Well sped their errand; with a patriot zeal
They spread the blessing for their country's weal.
                                              —Robert Bloomfield

"I am much gratified at the good sense manifested by the Cherokee Indians," Edward Jenner remarked in 1802. "Who would have thought that vaccination would already have found its way into the wilds of America?"[1] The Cherokees, it seemed, had the good fortune at an early date to benefit from a revolutionary medical advancement, the purposeful insertion of cowpox into an individual's body to give that person lasting immunity from smallpox. The indigenous nation's supposed vaccination became echoed in the May 1803 edition of London's *Gentleman's Magazine*, which reported that Cherokee leaders had heard "that the Great Spirit had gifted a white man, over the great water, with a power to prevent the smallpox." They reportedly asked Pres. Thomas Jefferson about this lifesaving breakthrough, received cowpox, and carried it as well as instructions on how to administer it back to their nation. *Gentleman's Magazine* affirmed, "It is a pleasing reflection that these untutored savages have spread it throughout their country, and that they are eminently expert in the practice of the new inoculation."[2] The English poet Robert Bloomfield perpetuated the belief in the Cherokees' early vaccination. As a footnote to his 1804 poetic tribute to Jenner, he identified those chiefs who sought "the white man and his bounteous God" as those of the Cherokee Nation.[3]

It would seem then our story now comes to an end. With access to cowpox and knowledge of how to administer it, Cherokees needed not worry about having another major epidemic of smallpox. They would not have understood the biological reasons why vaccination worked and for that matter neither did Jenner, the man credited with perfecting the procedure and making its value known to the wider world. Unknown to anyone at the time, cowpox infection—typically a minor skin disease that frequently passed from cows to dairy workers—stimulated a person's immune system to create antibodies that protected one from the cowpox virus's genetically similar cousin, smallpox. Jenner, to be sure, was not the first to identify cowpox as a preventative. Farmers in rural England had observed for some time that dairymaids who contracted the bovine skin illness never came down with smallpox, even after being exposed to the deadly human disease. A dairymaid relayed such information to Jenner in 1770 and the English farmer Benjamin Jetsy vaccinated his wife and two sons in 1774. Jenner, however, conducted a series of experiments that proved the efficacy of vaccine, and his 1798 publication *An Inquiry into the Causes and Effects of the Variolae Vaccinae* provided enough proof to convince learned men and world leaders that a solution to one of humankind's most dangerous diseases had been discovered. Following his inaugural publication, appeals to Jenner to send vaccine arrived from a variety of different places, and the practice of vaccination spread quickly, being introduced in the Austro-Hungarian Empire in 1799, France and the United States in 1800, Russia in 1801, and India in 1802.[4] The Cherokee Nation then, if Jenner is to be believed, was among the first nations to fight *Variola* with the lifesaving prophylactic of cowpox.

Our story does not come to such a quick and abrupt ending, however. President Jefferson did introduce vaccine to visiting Natives in the winter of 1801–1802, but these individuals were not who Jenner thought they were; the Cherokee Nation did not send a delegation to Washington, D.C., at that time, and no evidence indicates that they had any of their members vaccinated for another four years. Instead,

Ohio Valley and Great Lakes groups sent representatives, and they became the first indigenous peoples to be vaccinated. Jenner got his Natives mixed up when he learned of the momentous event in a letter written to him by the Boston physician, Benjamin Waterhouse. Waterhouse supplied Jefferson with the vaccine, which then became part of a larger gift of "civilization" that United States leaders aimed to bestow on Natives. The American physician explained to his English colleague, "Washington, Adams, and Jefferson have done everything to civilize that shrewd people." This benevolence included giving them ploughs, looms, spinning wheels, and "every common utensil in husbandry" as well as instructions in horticulture and herding. When "a grand embassy of certain tribes" arrived in Washington, D.C., in December 1801, Jefferson moved the efforts to introduce Euro-American culture into the realm of medicine. The president told the embassy's leader, Little Turtle, that the "GREAT SPIRIT had lately made a precious donation to the enlightened white men over the great water, first to a single person, and from him to another on this side [of] the waters, and then explained to him the history of the cow or kine-pock as a gift from heaven to preserve them from the smallpox, and even to banish it from the earth." Little Turtle consented to vaccination as did nine or ten of his warriors. They left the capital with live vaccine and instructions in how to administer it to their people. Jenner either thought Little Turtle, whose identity as a Miami chief was not revealed in Waterhouse's letter, was a Cherokee or inferred that Cherokees were among the "grand embassy."[5]

Our story then ends sometime later than 1802. The first known vaccinations of Cherokees occurred in 1806, although likely to a rather limited number and not enough to stop the spread of smallpox that year. A much more extensive and effective vaccination effort took place eighteen years later. In 1824 a smallpox scare sparked a round of vaccination that squelched an epidemic. This end to the story occurred in part along the lines that Jenner and his peers imagined: champions of Euro-American "civilization"—Protestant missionaries rather than the president in this case—brought the new medicine into the indigenous nation, vaccinated Natives, and gave them instructions on how to transmit cowpox to others. Cherokees then harvested the pus from their vaccinated kinsmen and passed it on to others who needed the lifesaving protection it provided. This development also occurred in a way contrary to Jenner and his peers' expectations. Vaccination was envisioned as part of a larger gift from enlightened and "civilized" Euro-Americans, whose culture would come to fully supplant that of indigenous peoples. Cherokees, however, came to pursue a pluralistic approach to healing and disease prevention over the course of the early nineteenth century. Vaccine and other Euro-American techniques and substances served as options for meeting one's healthcare needs, but Native beliefs and rites remained viable and strong through the 1820s and beyond. Cherokee medicine and its practitioners in other words proved resilient and vital and would not be displaced by the supposedly inevitable triumph of Euro-American culture.

• • • •

On the surface Cherokees appeared to rapidly and thoroughly adopt Euro-American culture during the early nineteenth century. War with Americans, punitive treaties that required massive land cessions, and the expansion of Euro-American settlement into former hunting grounds brought a collapse to the deerskin trade. Hunting gave way to livestock herding as the most important economic activity for Cherokee men, and the booming cotton plantations of the American South provided a ready market for beef, pork, leather, and draft horses. Cherokee women meanwhile eagerly took to cloth production. This new economy especially took off among Cherokees dislocated by the American Revolution. They had moved south and west into southeastern Tennessee, northwestern Georgia, and northeastern Alabama. Euro-American Loyalists and adopted American captives, moreover, composed a significant portion of their rebuilt communities; intermarriages had occurred; and a sizeable bicultural and bilingual minority emerged. Their communities became increasingly dispersed as families moved considerable distances from town centers in order to maximize grazing range for their animals. Some Cherokees even acquired African Americans as chattel slaves and had them tend to their growing livestock herds and even in some cases work cotton fields. Some communities to be sure changed more dramatically than others. The Valley Towns of the Hiwassee River's tributaries generally remained more compact and contained fewer numbers of intermarried Euro-Americans, bicultural offspring, and African American slaves, but these communities too could no longer live in nucleated villages as they also relied on livestock and had to disperse to find enough grazing land for their animals. In no way, though, did the Valley Towns represent one side of a bifurcated Cherokee Nation, one in which poor, monolingual, subsistence farmers stood in opposition to wealthy, bicultural, commercially oriented slaveholders. These two archetypes instead occupied two ends of a spectrum of diverse Cherokee communities.[6]

The federal government actively encouraged the Cherokees' cultural transition. Burdened by the cost of war with Natives, George Washington's administration—most notably his secretary of war Henry Knox—appointed agents to various tribes to instruct them in agriculture. The federal government would also support the work of Protestant missionaries, who would open schools near Native communities, teach farming and other vocational skills, offer English-language training, and endeavor to win converts to Christianity. Policy makers predicated this transformation on the belief that indigenous peoples' low rung of social development—that of "savagery" or "barbarity"—could be elevated to a "civilized" level by giving up hunting and adopting farming and herding. The architects of the "civilization" policy of course overlooked the fact that many Native women, particular Eastern Woodlands groups such as the Cherokees, farmed and had done so for hundreds of years before Europeans had arrived. The federal efforts thus entailed a transformation of gender roles; men would move out of the forests and into the fields, and women would move from the fields and into the homes, where they would dedicate themselves to spinning, weaving, and other household-centered chores. In the process, Natives would give up their no longer needed hunting grounds in exchange for breeding stock, farm equipment, spinning looms, and other items. Indigenous peoples would essentially disappear as their land base shrunk; as they assimilated into the general American populous as English-speaking, Christian farmers; and as they intermarried with Euro-Americans.[7]

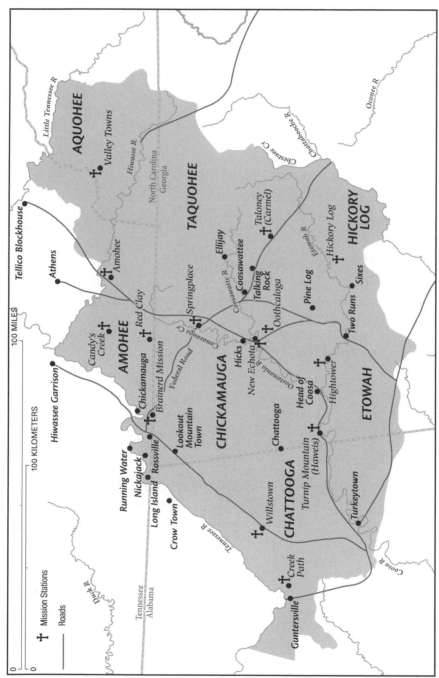

The Cherokee Nation after the revolution. Map by Darin Grauberger and Meghan Kelly, University of Kansas Cartographic Services.

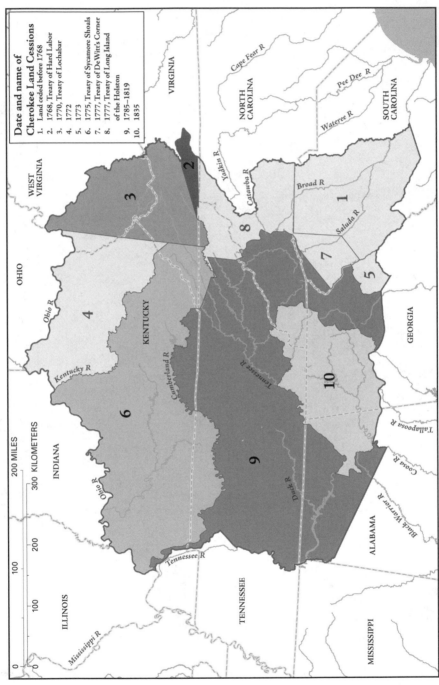

Cherokee land cessions prior to 1824. Map by Darin Grauberger and Meghan Kelly, University of Kansas Cartographic Services.

Date and name of
Cherokee Land Cessions
1. Land ceded before 1768
2. 1768, Treaty of Hard Labor
3. 1770, Treaty of Lochabar
4. 1772
5. 1773
6. 1775, Treaty of Sycamore Shoals
7. 1777, Treaty of DeWitt's Corner
8. 1777, Treaty of Long Island
    of the Holston
9. 1785–1819
10. 1835

The "civilization" plan of course did not work exactly how its supporters had hoped. Cherokees certainly did not disappear amid an enveloping tide of Euro-Americans. The indigenous nation's population in fact substantially increased from the end of the American Revolution. In 1809, the U.S. agent Return J. Meigs conducted a census in which the total number of Cherokees—excluding 583 freed and enslaved African Americans and 341 white residents—reached 12,395 individuals.[8] To this number, approximately 1,000 Cherokees, who had moved by then to Missouri and Arkansas, can be added, bringing the total to a reasonable population estimate of 13,395.[9] These over 13,000 Cherokees certainly represented more members of the nation than they had in 1783. One of course cannot know the extent of this population growth because data from the end of the revolution does not exist, but if Peter Wood's figure of 7,500 Cherokees in 1790 is correct, then the Cherokee population grew by 79 percent in a matter of one generation.[10]

Multiple variables factor into the increase of Cherokee population in the early nineteenth century. Vaccinations in 1806 helped their nation sustain growth by retarding the impact of smallpox in that year, and this story will be detailed later in this chapter. But, other factors certainly played consequential roles. The first and most obvious is the general peace that Cherokees enjoyed with their American and Native neighbors. Secondly, Cherokees incorporated a significant number of Euro-American Loyalists and other refugees from the American Revolution. Given the high death toll of Cherokee men during the revolution, the incorporation of men from the outside gave Cherokee women more possible marriage partners and helped them rebound relatively quickly from the demographic shock that successive American invasions had caused. Bicultural offspring were counted fully as Cherokees in the 1809 census. Third, fertility increased as Cherokees went through the transition to a livestock-based economy. As settled agriculturalists, Cherokee women had high rates of fertility in comparison to indigenous women from hunting and gathering tribes. Still hunting remained an essential component during the colonial era and this activity led men to be away from their villages for long periods of time, thus decreasing opportunities for couples to conceive. Herding kept men closer to home, while at the same time

providing a more consistent source of protein. The bilingual Cherokee Charles Hicks in fact identified this last variable as key to his
people's remarkable growth. "While they lived in their old way,"
Hicks explained about his ancestors, "moving from one place to place
in search of game through the whole winter, thus exposing their
women & children to many privations & hardships their numbers
were constantly diminishing: but since they have provided homes
for their women & children, where they can be warm & have enough
to eat the whole year, they are increasing like the white people."[11]
Hicks of course ignored women's work in his explanation; in most
Cherokee families, women defied the "civilization" plan and continued to do what they had done for hundreds of years—cultivate
corn, beans, and squash, which provided the bulk of the calories that
their families consumed.[12] That they could do this without the prospect of being captured by an enemy or without fear that the fruits
of their labor would be wiped out by a marauding army was essential
to the demographic growth of their families, clans, and nation. In
any event, Cherokee leaders expressed pride in their nation's population resurgence, used this fact to counter claims that Natives were
destined to disappear, and cited it as a reason why they could no
longer give up any more land.[13]

Another development that did not correspond with the aims of the
"civilization" policy was that the Cherokees grew more reluctant to
surrender any more land and melt into the larger American body poli-
tic, especially as they became more united under the leadership of a
cadre of commercially successful and generally bilingual ranchers,
planters, and slaveholders. By the early 1800s, Cherokee towns and
divisions sent representatives to a governing National Council, which
met annually. By 1808, the National Council began to keep record of
its decisions in written English and enforce their laws with a police
force known as the Lighthorse brigade. Among these laws were those
that asserted national control over selling land and made it illegal for
anyone to cede territory to the United States without approval of the
Cherokee government. Punishment for breaking this law brought
the death penalty. In 1819, Cherokees established their capital at the
junction of the Coosawattee and Conasauga Rivers and later named
it New Echota in honor of the old beloved town of Chota, which

then lay on ceded land. Ultimately, centralization efforts led to a written constitution in 1827 that created a three-tiered government of a principal chief, a National Council of two houses, and a judiciary. While modeled on the United States' example, this constitution exerted what the civilization policy had never envisioned: Cherokees wanted to remain apart from the larger American republic, keep their land base intact, and retain their status as a sovereign nation.[14]

Lastly, and most importantly for the purposes of understanding how Cherokees responded to vaccine, Protestant Christianity did not take root as quickly and as extensively as missionary organizations had hoped, and even among many nominal Native Christians, traditional beliefs and customs remained strong. Christianity to be sure made inroads. Cherokees became perhaps the most proselytized indigenous group of the early nineteenth century as representatives from a variety of denominations flooded into their nation. In general Cherokee leaders welcomed the missionaries because they promised to open schools and teach Native children English and other valuable skills. In 1802, the Moravians—a pietistic sect of German origins from nearby Salem, North Carolina—established a school for Cherokee children. Called Springplace, the school stood near the plantation of James Vann, a bicultural man, who before his death in 1809 amassed a fortune through his ferry business, ranching, slave trading, merchandizing, and commercial agriculture. The Moravians remained a small but continuous presence and in doing so educated a significant number of Cherokee students, including children belonging to several wealthier families such as the Vanns, Hicks, Ridges, and Waties. The Presbyterian minister Gideon Blackburn worked in the Cherokee Nation from 1804 until 1809, during which time he operated two schools in southeastern Tennessee one of which educated John Ross, who grew up to give his nation effective leadership in the 1820s and ultimately become the Cherokee Nation's longest serving principal chief (1828–66). Under the sponsorship of the well-funded, Boston-based American Board of Commissioners for Foreign Missions (ABCFM), Presbyterians returned to the Cherokee Nation in 1817 along with their Congregationalist partners. ABCFM Missionaries built schools and churches that ultimately functioned in nearly all districts of the Cherokee Nation, except the Valley Towns. This district hosted missionaries of a different sort. Various Baptist ministers visited there in the 1810s and 1820s, with Evan Jones of the Philadelphia-based Baptist Foreign Mission Board having the most important influence. He arrived in 1821, ran a school, and remained active among the Cherokees into the 1830s and beyond. Methodists had perhaps the most extensive influence throughout the entire nation, although given their highly decentralized administrative structure and that many of their ministers kept no records there is not as much known about their activities. Methodist camp meetings certainly occurred by the early 1820s and thereafter reoccurred on a regular basis, as circuit riders attracted diverse crowds drawn to the raucous, emotionally laden revivals. Still, only a small percentage of Cherokees became full members of Christian denominations. By the end of the 1820s, the various denominations counted only 1,399 members, with the Moravians having 45, ABCFM 167, Baptists 99, and Methodists 1,028.[15]

• • • •

For those who committed themselves to Christianity and for the thousands who chose not to do so, medicine proved to be a crucial concern. Cherokees did in general express a willingness to incorporate new substances and techniques from the outside world, and they saw missionaries as a possible option for healthcare. This should not be surprising. As men and women who dealt with spiritual matters, missionaries were looked upon as individuals who should attempt to cure and prevent illness. Ministers found themselves as having to practice medicine. They consequently used such opportunities to condemn Cherokee practitioners and promote Christianity. Most Cherokees, though, had no inclination to turn exclusively to Christianity. They instead forged a pluralistic society, one in which missionaries could be turned to in times of need while at the same time retaining a preference for Native practitioners as a healthcare option. Cherokees in other words adopted elements of Euro-American culture on their own terms.

Missionaries had a variety of techniques and substances they could offer Native patients based on what was still a premodern understanding of the body and disease. Nineteenth-century Euro-Americans generally believed that illness resulted when the body's four fluids or "humors"—blood, phlegm, yellow bile, and black bile—became out of balance or did not flow in the proper way. Toxins from the atmosphere or those passed from person to person were thought to produce this imbalance, as were sudden changes such as those caused by the weather or movement into a new area. Treatment was aimed to draw off excess humors, to remove blockages that prevented the movement of fluid, and to induce the evacuation of toxins. Thus vomiting, purging, bleeding, and blistering techniques, which sound rather odd to us today, made sense to nineteenth-century Americans. Euro-Americans at that time also took a variety of substances that were thought to assist the body in regaining balance. These included home remedies made from herbs and other natural substances known to be emetics, laxatives, or pain relievers. A variety of drugs could also be purchased. These included quite toxic mercury-based medicines such as calomel, which in low doses induced salivation and in larger doses served as a laxative. The drug produced side effects such as sore gums, loosening of the teeth, and liver damage. Laudanum was another major drug available for purchase. An opium-based substance, it alleviated pain and controlled coughing, making it especially useful for those suffering through the common chronic disease of tuberculosis. The most effective and less toxic drug in the nineteenth-century medicine chest actually had an indigenous origin: quinine. Made from a tree indigenous to the Andes and commonly referred to as Peruvian bark, quinine substantially ameliorated the symptoms of malaria by attacking the parasite in an infected individual's bloodstream and preventing it from reproducing. Euro-Americans of course did not understand at the time why these drugs produced the effects they did. Instead, they viewed them within the humoral theory as inducing the body to regain its natural balance of fluids. Thus, even the excruciating symptoms of calomel were seen as evidence that toxins were being shed, that the medicine was working, and that the body would in the end return to equilibrium.[16]

The Cherokees' sustained experience with Euro-American medicine began with the arrival of the Moravians in the early 1800s. The records of the Springplace mission are filled with numerous examples of Cherokees asking them for help. The Vann family in particular called on their German-American neighbors, who came to their assistance with thirty-two different medicinal plants they grew in their garden and a variety of drugs that they acquired from nearby Euro-American merchants or doctors.[17] The Moravians reputation as healers had spread beyond the Vanns' plantation, and Cherokees from a variety of different backgrounds sought them out for aid.[18] Young Wolf, for example, approached John and Anna Gambold, who oversaw Springplace from 1805 until 1821, for help with a fever that had troubled him for some time. "We gladly gave him some of the herbs that we had used for our children," the Gambolds recorded.[19] Similarly, Gunrod, who suffered from tuberculosis, came to the Moravians after consulting with an itinerant Euro-American doctor. The doctor prescribed elecampane roots, which Gunrod learned the Gambolds had on hand. The missionaries found it "a true joy" to fill the ill man's prescription.[20]

Moravians had many more opportunities to experience this joy. On a particular day in 1810, for example, they offered the old chief Koychezetel some advice about a bad eye that he could barely see out of, while later that evening they gave some herbs to another Native whose father had "black gout."[21] Some Cherokees traveled to Springplace on behalf of sick relatives at home. Otterlifter, for example, asked the Gambolds for advice on treating his "very sick and weak little child." The missionaries claimed "we helped as well as we could."[22] The former student George Hicks came back to his school in 1817 for "advice and medicine" to take to his ill father William.[23] The following year, "a very upstanding Indian" with a consumptive brother at home came to the Moravians and "asked humbly for the good medicine" that helped another Cherokee, Peggy Vann Crutchfield, to an apparent recovery from tuberculosis. Crutchfield, the Moravians' first convert, likely received an opium-based drug such as laudanum, and her recuperation under the Moravians' care had "been reported far and wide."[24] It may have been the same remedy that led David Watie to bring his consumptive neighbor Mouse to Springplace for aid. The Gambolds "gladly" offered him medicine.[25]

In some cases, Cherokees clearly sought out Moravians as an option when Native practitioners could not bring them relief. Edmund Falling, for example, brought his sick wife to Springplace in 1806 with "an illness that no one whose advice has been sought has really understood." The Gambolds declined to treat her because they too did not know what to do for her, but they did agree to treat others that had first visited Cherokee healers.[26] Suakee, for example, had seen a practitioner in his home community of Coosawatee for "pains in his side & fever" yet his treatment had no effect. Suakee's brother then traveled to Springplace for help. The missionaries at first proved reluctant, but they relented and provided some herbs. Suakee supposedly found some relief in this prescription and asked the Gambolds for more when his condition returned. Eventually, though, nothing could be done, and the man succumbed to his illness one year after receiving the Moravians' medicine.[27] In another instance, the parents of one of Springplace's students stopped by the school "on the way to an Indian doctor." They had been sick for "a long time" and decided to request help from the Gambolds as well. The missionaries provided them "some herbs."[28] The mother returned about two years later for further aid. The Moravians recorded, "She has already been sickly for a good while and has been under treatment by an Indian doctor who is also a conjuror. Instead of improving, however, she continues to get weaker. She fled to us since she could no longer endure it." The missionaries again gave her herbs and advice that the woman promised to take.[29]

Some Cherokees went in the opposite direction. Parents of Springplace students frequently preferred that their children receive Native medicine. In 1809, for example, two school boys came down with severe fevers. The children's fevers worsened, and a grandfather of one of the sick boys came and treated them both with roots that he gathered nearby that served as an emetic. The grandfather was satisfied that his prescription would work, but he did not reject the Moravian's medicine altogether. Upon his departure, he asked the Gambolds to share some of their medicinal herbs, which they gladly did. For their part, the missionaries appeared open-minded to the grandfather's practice as well and delighted that his medicine restored the two boys to health.[30] In another case, the Gambolds recorded with little commentary a case in which Tyger took his son Dawzizi home when he had a "strong influenza." A month later Dawzizi returned healthy, claiming that he had been treated by an "old Indian doctor," who scratched him with gar's teeth, rubbed the scars with a "juice of certain herbs," and extracted "a little horn of blood" from his body.[31] Tyger again withdrew one of his sons from school amid an epidemic. During a measles outbreak in 1822, the father took his son Pelican home to recover from the disease. He returned a couple of months later in full health.[32]

Similarly, a mother named Dawnee came to retrieve her "seriously ill" son George so that he could be treated, according to the Gambolds, in "the heathen way." The missionaries believed that such treatment had turned George against them. He returned with a "wild look" and had "completely changed in a troubled way." The Moravians eventually dismissed him for bad behavior.[33] Some parents brought practitioners with them to visit their children at Springplace. After discovering that one mother had done this, the Gambolds recorded in their journal that "such things happen from time to time but are kept very secret from us so that we find out about it only accidently." The Gambolds dismissively concluded that the parent tried to justify her actions "as if she were a rational mother."[34]

What was rational for the Moravians of course was that Cherokees reject the beliefs and rites of their customary medicine and adopt Christianity. They consequently used appeals for healthcare to discredit Native practitioners and promote their own religious beliefs. When Goadi of Chickamauga accepted their treatment after finding no relief from a Native practitioner, she not only received herbs but also "the truth from God's word."[35] In another case, the Gambolds rejoiced that one of their ill students did not go home when his brother was sent to fetch him. The trip home, they believed, would be too much of an ordeal and worse he would be delivered into "heathen hands." It was best, they concluded, that Jesus would "treat them according to his love."[36] Christianity was also the prescription for Gunrod. The Moravians gave him the elecampane roots he asked for and also a sermon, informing him that his life and health were in God's hands and he should "throw himself as a child into the arms of the Creator and Redeemer and ask Him that He Himself would bring him into His will."[37] The Gambolds became more forceful in the case of their student Jack, whose mother Qualiyuga attempted to take him home "to have spells cast over him." Moravians refused to let him go and had Peggy Crutchfield explain to the mother the "futility" of what she planned on doing. Qualiyuga subsequently left without her son and with much "displeasure."[38]

Whether Jack wanted to go went unrecorded, but in a similar incident the Moravians' influence over a female student ignited a cultural conflict over medicine within her family. In 1820, Tuhsiwal-liti came to Springplace to take his daughter Nancy home because, according to the Gambolds, "the grandmother had ordered a conjurer to protect her granddaughter against illnesses." Nancy did not want to go home and the Moravians were faced with the difficult position of neither wanting to anger the father nor exposing the girl to "heathenism." The Moravians decided that "we had to persuade her just to go with her father that she would not be forced to submit herself to the trickery." Nancy indeed resisted. She volunteered to care for her ill grandmother instead of joining her family in the Going-to-Water ceremony. When her brother came back to relieve her of caring for the elderly woman, Nancy ran back to Springplace.[39] Nancy later was baptized and helped persuade her father to become a Christian as well. She had no luck with her uncle Cananthoah, however. She condemned him for "carrying out magic in her house," and in return he allegedly threatened to kill her. The rest of the family took Nancy's side and chased the uncle away.[40]

The Moravians' converts in fact took the attack on Native medicine more directly to its practitioners and adherents. Charles Hicks led the way. Hicks had elevated his stature over the first couple of decades of the nineteenth century. In 1808 he not only refused the bribes that American agents had given his countrymen to sell a large quantity of their hunting grounds but he also publicly denounced those who had been bought off. In 1813, he became treasurer of the Cherokee Nation and in 1817 he became second principal chief. The Cherokees accorded Hicks a great deal of respect for his staunch dedication to preserving their lands and their political sovereignty, but at the same time he embraced Christianity and did not hide his skepticism of Native medicine. Since his youth, he suffered terribly from an ulcerated leg that at times flared up so badly that he could not walk. His condition was likely a manifestation of tuberculosis known as scrofula, for which he had continually sought out advice and treatment from Euro-American doctors.[41] He may or may not have consulted Native practitioners in his youth—he left no record that he had—but in any event he came to distrust them as an adult. He joined the Moravians in 1813 and immediately worked inside and outside of his own family to convince others to follow the Gospel.

Hicks's success was mixed at best. His immediate and much of his extended family converted to Christianity, but he made much less headway with Cherokee leaders with whom he had open conversations about medical practices and spiritual beliefs. In the same year he joined the Moravians he tried to convince the non-English speaking First Principal Chief Pathkiller and another prominent man known as Gu'ulisi about the futility of "the so called magic arts of the Indians." Hicks claimed that Native practitioners were "not in a position either to keep themselves healthy or to prolong their lives . . . that they are no more in a position to help others." Hicks concluded that "humans were not made just for this short life" but instead could be saved by Jesus and go to heaven.[42] Three years later, Hicks resumed his discussion with Gu'ulisi, and according to the Moravians, he encouraged the man to seek salvation through Jesus: "He asked him whether he could believe that a conjuror's immersing a man into water could protect him from sickness or could save a man from death when he saw how many people got sick often and also died regardless of these tricks." Gu'ulisi remarked that he still did not understand what Hicks was talking about and remained committed "for the time being to remain with the *ancient beliefs*."[43] Gu'ulisi would reject Christianity for the rest of his life, even to the extent of expelling his converted wife from their home.[44] Similarly, Pathkiller adhered to Native practices for the rest of his life. The principal chief remained generally tolerant of missionaries because they could teach the younger generation of Cherokees to speak English and other valuable skills, but he did not believe that the acquisition of those skills had to come at the expense of abandoning the beliefs and practices that had sustained his nation for so long.[45]

• • • •

Presbyterians and Congregationalists who worked for the ABCFM also had much difficulty overcoming Cherokee adherence to their own practitioners. They arrived from New England in 1817 with a high degree of certainty of their cultural superiority and optimism that Natives would readily accept Christianity. They first established Brainerd Mission, a boarding school on Chickamauga Creek, and then branched out from there. By 1824, the ABCFM organization had over a dozen ministers, teachers, and staff members along with their families tending to not only Brainerd but also stations at Taloney, Creek Path, Willstown, Hightower, and Turnip Mountain. As happened with the Moravians, the newly arrived missionaries found themselves administering healthcare to Cherokees, doing so to promote Christianity, and yet having little success in displacing Native medicine.

ABCFM ministers met requests to practice medicine with varying enthusiasm. Ironically, the only one who had any formal medical training, Elizur Butler, felt most overwhelmed, incompetent, and reluctant to tend to healthcare needs. He had spent a year training to be a physician before taking up his calling as a missionary, and his colleagues referred to him as "Doctor" despite his own self-doubts. Cherokees also looked upon him as a physician and called upon him to relieve them of various ailments.[46] He often agreed to do so, yet complained to his colleagues that medical duties meant he spent most of his time with more affluent Natives rather than the poorer, non-English speakers whose souls he believed were in most need of the Gospel. "I have ever been sorry that the title of Doctor was palmed on me in the manner it was; and have feared and still fear it may prove a disadvantage to the cause," Butler complained.[47] His ABCFM colleagues encouraged him to persevere in medicine and he did so. During the summer of 1822, he spent most of his time with ill Cherokees, administering treatment such as bleeding and prescribing a variety of drugs from the Euro-American pharmacopeia.[48]

The fate of one of those patients gave Butler and his colleagues confidence that Western medicine and Christian theology would serve the Cherokees much better. In early June 1822, the converted and bilingual Charles Reece called upon Butler to visit a sick woman, who suffered from what her neighbors considered an "incurable" condition. Exactly what Butler did for the woman went unrecorded, but his fellow missionaries claimed that Christian medicine "had the desired effect, & being administered under [Butler's] direction for some time she had so far recovered as to ride abroad."[49] They also added that his treatment left her "much better and in a hopeful way to recover" and applauded his effort to "prescribe for her spiritual maladies" as well.[50] Apparently, she and some of her family members believed that Butler did not do enough. She went through a Going-to-Water ceremony sometime after his initial visit. By the end of June her condition deteriorated and she died on July 2. ABCFM missionaries, unquestionably confident in whatever Butler had prescribed, concluded that Cherokee medicine had to be at fault, claiming she "had fallen a victim to her imprudence; or perhaps to the mistaken notions of her relatives." They added that "nothing could have been more injudicious" than "the Indian methods of curing the sick . . . in a case like hers."[51]

Yet Butler still wondered whether medicine was the best use of his time. "I knew not that I should ever be employed in a heathen land as a physician," he complained to his governing board. "If it is wished that I should practice medicine, I would say I have at present little or no time to study, and am constantly lacking in the knowledge of some disorders." He believed he needed more training and worried that he would become discredited because of his lack of skill.[52] Appeals to him to practice his medical craft nonetheless continued. Despite some failures, his confidence gradually grew. In March 1823, for example, he visited a sick Cherokee man several times and led his colleagues to believe that the "prescriptions" he gave provided the man "great" relief. The man, though, died soon after Butler left him. His colleagues exonerated Butler from any blame, claiming that the death resulted from the man eating a "large quantity of food" contrary to the doctor's order.[53] Butler gave more effective treatment the following fall. Then, he prescribed Peruvian bark to both children and adults around Brainerd and others who came to visit him with cases of malaria.[54]

Other missionaries with even less training had more confidence in their ability to use Euro-American medicine to further their cause. The Reverend John Elsworth, for example, found soon after arriving at his mission station at Turnip Mountain that Cherokees asked him for aid. He subsequently purchased a medical text and dictionary to consult in such cases. With this self-instruction, he diagnosed and treated a variety of illness, claiming to be successful in all cases. Such success he hoped would help turn Cherokees to Christ.[55] He reported back to the ABCFM's governing board: "In this country far from civilized society and consequently physicians a teacher must be called many times to visit the sick & dying." He claimed to have made twenty visits to ill patients within one year and added that "I think it a favorable circumstance, if we can gain the confidence of the people sufficiently to trust themselves in our hands in such occasions of danger, rather than apply to those called conjurors."[56]

The Reverend Moody Hall also had no formal medical training, but in 1819 he headed off to establish his station at Taloney with among other things medical books and an assortment of drugs including Peruvian bark, calomel, and laudanum.[57] He was not afraid to use them either. In July 10, 1822, for example, he sent a sick Cherokee student home. The boy's father appealed to the reverend to send medicine, which Hall promptly did by sending an emetic. Soon thereafter, Hall received the frightful message that the boy had died, prompting him to go to the family. He was relieved to find that the boy had only fainted, but of course could not know that the medicine he prescribed probably caused the boy to pass out. The vomiting that followed a dose of emetic almost certainly led to dehydration. A few days after Hall had made his prescription, the boy remained sick, leading the minister to encourage the family to look to the Judeo-Christian spirit world for comfort and aid. He preached to the family and led them in prayers.[58]

It is not clear whether the boy improved thereafter, but Hall certainly continued to look for such opportunities to spread the Gospel. Less than two months later, for example, "an urgent request" reached him to visit two adult male members of a family stricken with a high fever. He had to decline due to other obligations and the next day learned that the two men died. Hall recorded in his journal: "I sincerely regret that I cannot attend to such calls. By visiting the sick & distressed the religion of Christ may be conveniently recommended."[59] He did find time on many other occasions, however.[60] Amid a whooping cough outbreak in the summer of 1823, for example, he spent part of a day with his colleague Daniel Butrick "visiting the sick, & in giving such direction for the recovery of the soul, as well as the body, as we were able."[61] Prayers were undoubtedly part of the prescription that Hall gave to an "old Cherokee woman" who came to him from more than forty miles away "to seek relief from a distressing disease." In addition to Christ, Hall introduced her to "a course of mercury," which he recorded as being effective.[62] Hall's medicine was not always welcome of course. The missionary visited the home of one of the ABCFM's prized converts, Alexander Sanders, several times during the summer of 1823 and tried in vain to get permission from the Sanders family to treat one of their sick children. Objections came from Sanders's wife, whom Hall described as "being so much in favor with the old practice with the sick" that she "prevented my doing anything for the poor sick children."[63]

Hall also found that many Cherokees insisted on following "old" practices when it came to combatting a measles outbreak in May 1822. Hall and Cherokee converts such as David Brown and Alexander Sanders had spent a great deal of effort in preaching to residents of Taloney against the "wicked ways" of their ancestors.[64] When measles erupted among his students, however, Hall was shocked to learn that few attended one day because "a conjurer had called all the town together to conjure away the measles." From the minister's description, the rite that called his students away was a physic dance. To combat what he dismissed as "superstition," the minister held a meeting of Christian "enquirers," or those who attended his church and appeared to be moving toward baptism, but he made little headway even with them. Instead, he found that in general each enquirer wanted to keep one foot in Cherokee medicine as one foot stepped toward the new religion. "On finding all present & desirous for instruction, I was lead to hope that the spirit of God was really striving with them," he lamented. "But a short time since . . . [they] were among the first to attend all the frolics & foolish traditions of the country." Upon his chastisement, his congregation gave him the impression that "they appear anxious to know the will of God & say they have no more pleasure in their former ways."[65] The reverend learned later, though, that the local practitioner still had sway and convinced many that the measles outbreak had resulted because of the missionary's presence in Taloney and because some residents "had not faith in their old ways."[66]

ABCFM records indeed paint a picture of Cherokees not giving up their culture so easily and in many cases trying to forge a coexistence between the so-called old ways and Christianity. The experience of Beamer, a prominent Cherokee from the Hightower community, clearly exemplified this pluralism. In July 1822, Beamer oversaw the burial of a man from his community, an event that the Reverend William Chamberlain witnessed. On Beamer's cue, the women appeared to exclaim "Ahquatse" or "Oh my son" repetitively as others put the man into a coffin and buried him. Upon completion, Beamer invited Chamberlain to preach through his interpreter, the Cherokee convert John Arch. Chamberlain recorded, "I endeavored to explain to them how sin came into the world, and death by sin & exhorted them to repentance and faith in Jesus Christ." The message seemed to resonate with Beamer.[67] A year later Beamer and some of his community members had more extensive discussions with Daniel Butrick again through John Arch. Butrick wrote of Beamer: "This dear man seems peculiarly anxious for instruction. He wishes to be baptized." A day later, Butrick provided more information about Christianity and explained to them "what conduct was sinful." The minister did not provide specific details in his journal about what particular conduct, except that he "distinctly" explained the Ten Commandments.[68] Apparently, Beamer did not take to heart the first commandment. Beamer was baptized in 1824 but continued to participate in Cherokee customs conducted by Native practitioners, whose medicine revolved around paying respect to a variety of different spirits rather than a singular deity as Christianity demanded. Butrick gave Beamer a stern rebuke for such idolatry, and then a year later the minister felt compelled to suspend the Cherokee elder from the Hightower Church of Christ for his adherence to "ancient customs."[69]

Other Cherokees found the ABCFM's condemnation of their customs too much to bear. Mostly opposition to missionaries manifested itself in a passive manner. The majority simply and politely chose not to attend Christian services. At times, though, the animosity boiled over in confrontation. In April 1824, Moody Hall reported that a naked man burst into his home and threatened to kill him, his wife, and child. His Cherokee neighbors intervened and assisted in having the Lighthorse brigade arrest the man. Reverend William Potter believed his ABCFM colleague had exaggerated what happened and dismissed the attack as the act of a drunk man, who later apologized.[70] The incident nonetheless brought to light the animosity that the missionary presence at Taloney had created. Hall's condemnation of alcohol bred resentment among those who liked to drink, but his efforts to go beyond teaching basic skills to Taloney's children and his broader challenge to Cherokee customs divided the town. A report came to him that residents had grown upset with him because "I came to teach the children & have been teaching the old people & making fools of them." He particularly charged Taloney's head chief, a man closely tied with the organization of such rites as the physic dance that Hall had condemned in 1822, for being "unfriendly" and encouraging the attack on him and his family. Hall's wife, moreover, did little to ingratiate herself to the community. The reverend learned that Cherokees harbored some resentment toward her because she did not display proper hospitality. Her poor health—a fact that her neighbors may not have been fully aware of—kept her confined to her house and unable either to visit other households or welcome visitors into hers.[71]

Resentment towards the intrusive missionaries also manifested itself in other ways. In spring 1824, Chuleoa and other leading men of Hightower asked Pathkiller and Hicks to remove the ABCFM station from their community. Hightower's children complained about the care they received from their teachers but the community in general grew tired of them. "They are trying to do away [with] our common custom of meeting in our townhouse," Chuleoa and his peers charged. They added that "other strange rules they are adopting which appears to us ought not to be suffered."[72] These rules certainly involved prohibitions on physic dances and other rites designed to protect the health and well-being of Hightower's residents. Animosity toward missionaries also emerged in Willstown, the home of Pathkiller. The aged chief and his allies expressed strong opposition to the ABCFM during the summer of 1824, and he and his political allies appeared poised to use their influence in the upcoming National Council meeting to persuade their countrymen to expel the intrusive Presbyterians and Congregationalists.[73]

• • • •

By 1824 then a broad spectrum of Cherokees had experience with missionaries and their medicine. And, a pattern of pluralism regarding healthcare became established in their nation. Some Cherokees clearly showed a curiosity in what the missionaries had to offer in regard to the treatment of illness; for some this was an avenue for further exploration of Christianity and ultimate conversion; for others this was simply an effort to find what might work and not a sign that they had given up completely on their own medicine; for yet others Christianity was a foreign and corrupting element that ought to be resisted. The Cherokees' acceptance of vaccine fit this pattern of pluralism.

To reconstruct the Cherokees' experience with vaccine let us return to the early nineteenth century. In the summer of 1801 Benjamin Waterhouse sent Thomas Jefferson cowpox, and Jefferson immediately began experimenting on his family, slaves, and others who would consent to having the new procedure performed on them. Cherokees barely missed being among this early group. They held a series of talks with the president and Secretary of War Henry Dearborn from June 30 until July 10, 1801, but no evidence indicates that Jefferson experimented on them, and even if he did, the cowpox that the president had at his disposal arrived ineffective.[74] Vaccine indeed was difficult to send. Waterhouse received his supply from England since cowpox was not prevalent among American cattle herds. British physicians sent the matter in a dried state—on a cotton thread that was run through the skin lesion of a recently vaccinated individual. It took Jenner several tries to send the substance across the Atlantic since the live viruses of the bovine disease had a short shelf life. It could persist for about three months when kept at room temperature, but if exposed to high heat it could quickly become ineffective. Once receiving cowpox, Waterhouse could sustain it by continually vaccinating people and then harvesting the pus from those he infected. The Boston physician became a common source for the vaccine during the early 1800s, and Jefferson himself helped develop novel ways to ship it and keep it active.[75] In August 1801, Jefferson finally received effective matter and successfully administered it to nearly two hundred people in and around Monticello.[76] Thereafter, the president made it common practice to include vaccine and instructions in how to propagate it as part of his diplomacy with Natives, leading Jenner himself to believe that the procedure he championed was making its way into "the wilds of America."[77]

The first vaccinations of the Cherokees would not unfold as Edward Jenner imagined to have happened, however. The indigenous nation sent a large delegation to Washington, D.C., in December 1805 and their young interpreter—Charles Hicks—and possibly others submitted to vaccination.[78] Hicks hoped to transmit the lifesaving prophylactic back to his people, but he proved unable to do so. The Cherokee leader did not fully explain why, other than saying that he "lamented often that we were so careless that we did not preserve the kine pox [illegible] I was inoculated with."[79] He had reason to lament. Smallpox had beaten the delegation back to their nation and began spreading among Cherokee families in southeastern Tennessee.[80] There is little else known about how Cherokee practitioners responded to this particular epidemic, but they likely did what they had in the past and tried to avoid exposure, closed their communities off from the outside world, and practiced the smallpox ceremony. Such actions, however, occurred within a dramatically different context from that of the colonial era. Traffic through their nation had substantially increased with the rising affluence of Cherokee families engaged in commerce with nearby Euro-American communities and with a federal road carved through the middle of their nation that connected Knoxville, Tennessee, with Augusta, Georgia.[81] Their increasingly dispersed settlement patterns, moreover, had mixed consequences for leaders trying to protect their communities. On one hand, infections spread more slowly among a dispersed population with families living in the most remote areas having a greater chance of escaping exposure than they would have if they still lived in compact settlements. On the other hand, such living arrangements inhibited communication and made it difficult to enforce isolation of an entire community and quarantine of infected individuals. In other words, Cherokees could not control who came into and out of their communities to the degree that they once were able to do. In such a situation, vaccine would have an obvious benefit.

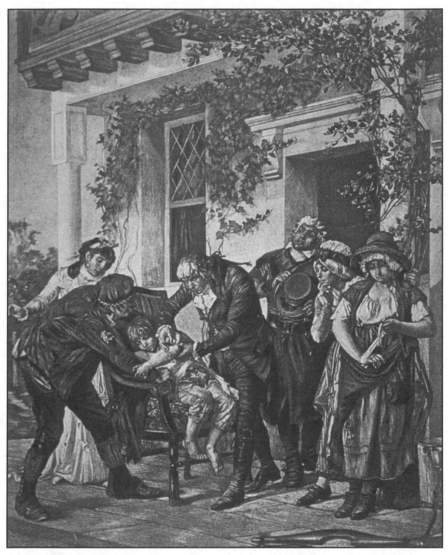

The First Vaccination—Dr. Jenner, photogravure by Georges-Gaston Mélingue (1894).
Edward Jenner has received immortal fame for championing a method that offered
certain protection from smallpox: the deliberate insertion of cowpox matter into an
incision on the arm. As with other substances and techniques from Western medicine, vaccination became one element of the Cherokees' pluralistic approach to
medicine. (Image courtesy of the History of Medicine Division at the National
Library of Medicine)

Cherokee leaders indeed pursued vaccine through other avenues. Pathkiller, then in his prime as one of his people's most prominent figures, crafted an appeal through his bilingual colleague John Lowery to the federal agent Return J. Meigs. They exclaimed, "Friend, the smallpox are spreading through nation. . . . Do Friend procure as quick as possible some of the cowpox & send it . . . without loss of time, we wish a doctor to come on also possibly some of the doctors of Knoxville or Maryville may be in possession of the matter if not procure it from the North by the post in complying with this request you will be instrumental in saving many lives."[82] Meigs sent a Dr. McNeel to them, but the Tennessee physician did not "think so favorably" of vaccine and instead advocated the older practice of variolation to which some Cherokee leaders objected.[83] McNeel was later paid $150 for his services, but it is unclear what exactly he did, if anything.[84]

Another appeal for vaccine reached Meigs through Daniel Ross, a Scottish merchant married to Mollie McDonald of the Bird Clan. Their son John had contracted smallpox before vaccine could arrive, leaving his distraught father to urge the federal agent to forward vaccine to protect those who had not yet been exposed. He relayed the information that Cherokee leaders did not want variolation but instead "preferred taking their chances till the kinepox could be brought into use, it being the kind that Pathkiller spoke for." "I must still think the [Cherokee] Nation will acknowledge with a grateful heart that you are the savior of many of them by its introduction," Ross added. He concluded that he would personally see to cowpox's circulation.[85] It would be too late for John Ross, of course, who nonetheless survived the frightful infection and grew up to become a chief to his people, but for others vaccine arrived in time. By June the epidemic seemed to subside at least in the portion of the Cherokee Nation around Gideon Blackburn's schools in southeastern Tennessee. Blackburn reported: "The small pox has been pretty fatal, but the introduction of vaccination has stopped its career so far as it has been practiced."[86]

How vaccine actually arrived and how extensively it became disseminated is not clear. Blackburn hoped to be the agent that introduced the lifesaving substance and procedure, but his efforts seem to have come up empty. He first inquired about the availability of cowpox in nearby Euro-American communities in Tennessee but found none. He then wrote to a missionary organization in Philadelphia, which agreed that vaccinated persons should immediately be sent into the Cherokee Nation along with a doctor who would teach Natives the procedure. The missionary board hoped the U.S. government would authorize such an effort, but no evidence suggests that federal agents did such a thing.[87] Blackburn's own students went unvaccinated, and most suffered through the disease.[88] Wherever vaccine came from, it did not get to families living along the Etowah River. The epidemic flared up there in the fall, and "many" reportedly became infected and died.[89] Among those who perished was John Vann, a former Chickamauga warrior who had avoided infection during the American Revolution only to succumb to the illness over twenty years later. His wife, Molly, and son suffered through the disease and survived.[90] However extensively vaccination was practiced, it did not arrest the spread of the epidemic. The year 1806 then could hardly be considered a watershed moment for the Cherokees and their ongoing fight against colonialism's most dreaded germ.

After 1806 some sporadic vaccinations of Cherokees occurred. Vaccine became increasingly accepted and available in the United States during the first two decades of the nineteenth century, and one can safely assume that some affluent Cherokees, especially those with African American slaves, readily sought out cowpox and had it administered to their family and all others on their plantations. Since these would have been private decisions and individually paid for, they would not have shown up in either public records of the United States or the Cherokee Nation. A more public episode of vaccination did show up in the documentary record. In February 1820, Dr. J. C. Strong of Knoxville administered cowpox to "a large number" of students at the ABCFM's Brainerd mission. Strong gave further instructions in how to pass the vaccine on to the remainder of the students. The missionaries originally failed to record this event when it happened yet made note of it some nine months later. Such initial omission raises the question that vaccination may have been commonplace wherever they organized schools and that they only brought it to the attention to the ABCFM governing board so that Strong would receive credit for his benevolence.[91] Perhaps Presbyterians and Congregationalists had disseminated vaccine in their other mission schools. If they had, such actions did not cause any recorded controversy.

More certainly, the year 1824 marks a watershed moment in the Cherokees' experience with *Variola*. In that year, a smallpox scare led to a significant wave of vaccination that effectively halted an epidemic. Smallpox had reportedly reached the Valley Towns in June.[92] According to one report, five Cherokees brought the disease with them on their return from Philadelphia, while another report indicated that a traveler from Kentucky inadvertently introduced the disease.[93] Cherokees had their own explanation of the disease's origin. With what was an apparent reference to the Uktena, Cherokees told the Moravians that "an unbelievably big snake brought this horrible pest in the Nation." The missionaries also learned that "it has a white head and is as thick as a human. Even its stench is supposed to be so unbearable that it kills people on the spot."[94] The children under Moravian care continued to think of the Uktena, even after attending Sunday services on June 20. Springplace's students reportedly "had their separate service" and prayed "from time to time to a large eagle and plead with him to keep illness away from them."[95] The children showed their awareness of their people's cosmology; an avian being was the appropriate countervailing spirit to call upon to destroy the snake-like Uktena. Perhaps they called upon Jesus as well.

Cherokee leaders turned to vaccine. In 1824, two men who had previously sought cowpox for their countrymen sat at the top of their national government, Pathkiller as principal chief and Charles Hicks as second principal chief. There is no reason to believe that either Hicks or Pathkiller changed his mind on vaccine, but by then John Ross had assumed much of the day-to-day responsibility for overseeing national business. Pathkiller had grown elderly, while Hicks remained incapacitated much of the time due to his health problems. Ross served as president of the National Council, had yet to commit to any particular Christian denomination, and was closely allied to Pathkiller.[96] During the first half of 1824, he led a delegation in Washington, D.C., then lobbying the federal government to fulfill its past treaty obligations. When he came home in June, he brought cowpox with him. It is unknown whether he heard reports of the outbreak on his way home or whether returning with smallpox vaccine was something regularly done. In any event, the matter that he had in his possession unfortunately did not arrive in an effective form.[97] Washington, D.C., was not the only source for cowpox, however. Euro-American doctors in nearby states provided an option and newspapers in both Georgia and North Carolina reported that vaccine had been requested from the Cherokee Nation.[98] Whether such efforts to procure cowpox proved fruitful is unknown, but what is known is that by 1824 Cherokee officials embraced vaccination and took efforts to secure its benefits for their people, even if they were not unanimous in their views on other aspects of Euro-American culture.

If ordinary Cherokees did not receive vaccine through the agency of their leaders, then they could seek it out from missionaries. After learning of the outbreak, Moravian minister Johann Schmidt wrote, "As soon as I received news of it, my first thought was to get 'cowpox' and to inoculate our children and as many people in the neighborhood here as were willing to have this done." He claimed to have convinced the Presbyterian minister Daniel Butrick about the propriety of taking such action.[99] Whether Schmidt's persuasion was necessary or not, Butrick decided to undertake the task. He inquired in many places in eastern Tennessee and rode as far as Knoxville, where he finally found a doctor that had cowpox in his possession. Butrick returned to the Cherokee Nation and reached Springplace on June 30, when he passed cowpox on to Cherokee students under Moravian care. The vaccine took and several days later the Moravians harvested cowpox matter from those vaccinated and passed it onto a variety of other people. By July 10, the Moravians claimed to have vaccinated a total of 130 individuals, and they continued this activity thereafter.[100] Before and after a church service the following day, they administered cowpox to "brown and black people [who] let themselves be inoculated."[101] The Moravians never indicated the final number that they vaccinated, only reporting that they were "able to inoculate a large number of Indians and Negroes."[102]

The full significance of the Moravians' efforts was not limited to what happened at Springplace but how vaccine became disseminated from there to a much larger number. Vaccinations that occurred at Springplace had the ripple effect that Edward Jenner had imagined

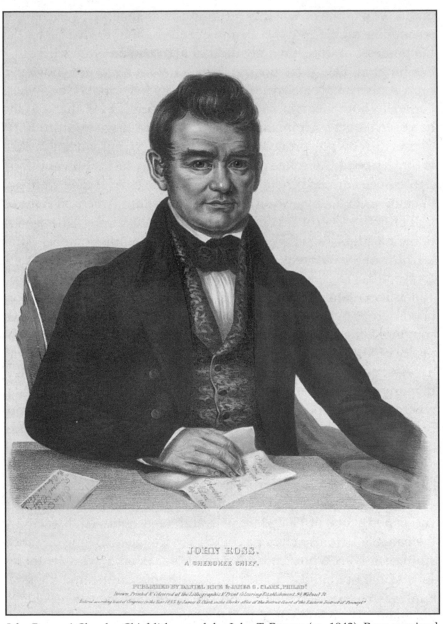

John Ross—A Cherokee Chief, lithograph by John T. Bowen (ca. 1843). Ross survived smallpox in his youth and as president of the Cherokee National Council sought to have his people vaccinated during the 1824 smallpox scare. (Courtesy of the Library of Congress, Prints and Photographs Division, LC-USZC4–3156)

had happened in the Cherokee Nation back in 1802. The Moravians recorded that people arrived at their mission "daily" to acquire vaccine and take it back to their families and communities.[103] These seekers came from varied backgrounds. The Christianized Hicks family of Oothcaloga acquired vaccine through Jay Hicks, son of the Moravian-convert William and nephew of Charles. Gardiner Greene then a fifteen-year-old student at Springplace also served as a vehicle for the dissemination of cowpox. He entered school back in 1819 at the age of ten with the name Young Wolf (not the same Young Wolf who had earlier sought help from the Gambolds for his fever) and had his new name bestowed upon him from the Moravians in honor of the Boston benefactor who paid his tuition. Greene was vaccinated during the 1824 smallpox scare and then traveled home to Coosawattee, where his father Mouse was a prominent resident. Mouse—the same individual who had shown up in 1817 at Springplace seeking help with his consumption—generally spoke highly of the Moravians, although he never sought them out for serious religious instruction.

Tyger of Big Spring also came to the Moravians for vaccine. Tyger had ten years earlier taken his son home from Springplace to receive Cherokee medicine for influenza, and at some point had become known to the Moravians as a "conjuror."[104] Now with smallpox lurking, he came to the Christians seeking their medicine. He took his son Pelican "home for a while, so that through him he can inoculate his family and the neighborhood there with cowpox." Such an action was certainly not a step toward embracing Christianity. Soon after the 1824 smallpox scare, the Tyger joined a movement known as White Path's Rebellion that among other things objected to the missionaries' interference with Native customs. Tyger, it seemed, did not have a problem accepting an aspect of Euro-American medicine that he thought would protect his family but did have a problem accepting the theology of those from whom he acquired it. His action indeed fit the larger pattern that developed in his Nation over the last couple of decades and undoubtedly exemplified the objectives of many of those who flocked to Springplace in July 1824. They sought out the aid and assistance of missionaries but did so with no intention of abandoning Cherokee beliefs and practices.

ABCFM missionaries also spread vaccine but did encounter some resistance. On July 7, Butrick carried cowpox to the Haweis Mission near the Hightower community, where the Reverend John Elsworth reported he would "probably" administer it to the children attending his school the next day. He did not record whether he did. Butrick also carried cowpox to Moody Hall's station at Taloney, but there the local practitioner gave the ABCFM ministers fits. After receiving news of the epidemic in June, the practitioner, who had two years earlier attempted to drive away the measles, now held a smallpox ceremony. The Moravians learned from their ABCFM colleagues that "at this dance, where all sorts of amazing trickery is carried out, a tea made of various herbs and roots is drunk. On such occasion the sorcerer prays to the black dog in the north, the white one in the east, the gray one in the south and the red one in the west. The sorcerer receives 7 deerskins for his art and from each family a string of corals."[105] The small number of Cherokee Christians, however, refused to attend. Rev. Moody Hall reported, "The Christians all say that they think more of a short sincere prayer than of their seven days fasting & drinking physic."[106] Hall of course would cast out any of his converts that tried to partake in both Christian and Cherokee rituals. After vaccine arrived, Hall attempted to convince the unconverted of the folly of their ways and induce them to accept vaccine. He recorded: "We had been to the expense & gratuitously offered to inoculate all that would come & by this man's opposition none would avail themselves of this safe preventive but the members of the church & their children."[107]

Their refusal to receive vaccine from Hall, however, does not mean they rejected cowpox in itself and does not mean that they failed to become vaccinated during the smallpox scare. Cherokees in general embraced a pluralistic approach to health and healing. Residents of Taloney probably would have and perhaps did accept vaccine from a friendlier source and saw no conflict between this and attending the smallpox ceremony conducted by their local practitioner. What they did have a conflict with was Hall's overbearing manner. The reverend had generated much hostility for his condemnation of Cherokee customs and lack of hospitality. Cherokees continued to express their opposition to this man through the summer. They told him that they had agreed to let him into their neighborhood for only five years, that his "time was pretty near up," and that his main offense had been that he had repetitively turned away people when they showed up at his door hungry.[108] Hall in other words had violated basic Cherokee custom, thus setting himself up as an outsider who did not have the best interest of his hosts at heart. Why would they accept his medicine? The smallpox ceremony, a rite based on community solidarity and reciprocity, seemed a better solution to the impending danger.

While opposition to Hall may have inhibited the administration of cowpox, a significant vaccination effort that encompassed a wide spectrum of the Cherokee Nation did occur and such an effort appears to have paid off. Smallpox never proliferated outside of the Valley Towns.[109] Even in this more remote area, the epidemic appeared to be short-lived. Why this was the case unfortunately cannot be known with certainty. Vaccinations may have occurred in this region, and residents there almost certainly resorted to strategies of avoidance, isolation, and quarantine. The individuals that were in the best position to report what actually happened did not provide posterity with much to go on, however. Reverends Thomas Dawson and Evan Jones staffed the Valley Town mission for the Baptist Foreign Mission Board. Little is known about their work before 1826, as correspondence before then does not survive except what became published in religious periodicals at the time. Only two letters dated to 1824 were published, one by Dawson on August 24 and another by Jones on December 2.[110] Neither mentions smallpox or vaccination efforts, or anything else that suggests a calamitous event had recently happened. Perhaps the Baptists had acquired cowpox for their small congregation, and the substance then became distributed to non-Christians. Perhaps, the preventative mechanisms of Cherokee medicine were enough to keep the epidemic contained among a relatively few families. Perhaps both worked together. One cannot know, and may never know, given the lack of source material. What remains certain, though, is that the epidemic fizzled out as the summer wore on, and unlike the 1806 outbreak, *Variola* neither spread nor became reintroduced to another region of the indigenous nation. In the end, vaccination helped make the 1824 outbreak only a scare and not a reality for the vast majority of Cherokees.

• • • •

The Cherokees' ancestors crafted useful strategies of avoidance, isolation, and quarantine to fight *Variola*, and then in 1824 descendants of those ancestors had the added protection of vaccine. The acceptance of this revolutionary medicine from the Western world, however, did not happen at the expense of Native medicine. Cherokees had established a pluralistic pattern when it came to healthcare, and vaccination fit within that context, even when missionaries had hoped that it and other drugs and procedures they introduced would discredit Native practitioners. Vaccine in other words may have been a gift from the "civilized" world to indigenous peoples, but contrary to the expectations of Jenner, Waterhouse, Jefferson, and others, Natives would adopt it on their own terms, as a supplement to a resilient indigenous medical culture that Cherokees, even many who professed Christianity, wanted to maintain as an option for their healthcare needs.

Missionaries indeed found that they could not easily displace such a belief system, and in fact many realized that they had to accommodate Cherokee medicine, if they were to add and keep converts. After 1824 Cherokee membership in Methodist churches quickly outpaced the ABCFM, Moravians, and Baptists because the former seemed unconcerned with how Cherokees sought healthcare. Moody Hall learned this the hard way. Following his condemnation of the smallpox ceremony, he feared losing one of his church members named Daniel, who had learned from other Cherokees that one could join the Methodists and "still go on as before."[111] Similarly William Chamberlain then stationed at Pathkiller's hometown of Willstown lamented that those willing to become Christians went to the Methodist because it was easier for them to join.[112] One Cherokee who took this supposedly easy route was John Ross. In October 1829, he joined the Methodist Church. Although Ross kept his motives quiet, one can guess that the savvy principal chief must have known that such a decision had political consequences. His Christianity marked him as a "civilized" leader in the eyes of sympathetic whites, particularly missionaries, who could use their political weight against other Americans bent on destroying Native sovereignty and expropriating their land, while his brand of Christianity reflected a pluralism in which Cherokee beliefs and practices would continue.[113]

Perhaps no one lamented this pluralism more than the Presbyterian Daniel Butrick. Following the 1824 smallpox scare, Butrick went on the offensive against Native practitioners, even going so far as to write a letter to Pathkiller explaining why Cherokee customs were wrong.[114] He made little headway with Pathkiller, a man who earnestly sought out vaccine for his people back in 1806 yet rejected Christian theology throughout his life. Butrick even lost ground with those who had converted, as the experience of Charles Moore of Hightower demonstrates. Moore, a man described as "half white" yet who spoke only Cherokee, submitted to baptism in 1824 and joined the ABCFM church. Three years later, however, he was also receiving instruction from a practitioner "in the art of conjuration." Rev. Isaac Proctor described this practitioner's medicine as "purely heathen as almost anything to be met with on the River Ganges. When conjuring, they pray to almost every creature such as white dogs, butterflies, turtles, etc. etc."[115] Proctor and Butrick consequently suspended Moore in 1827 and then readmitted him to church membership one year later after he supposedly agreed to give up Native medicine.

Yet Moore could not bring himself to commit himself and his family to one option for comfort and aid, as Butrick found out during one particularly volatile church service at Hightower. Most church members there, Butrick believed, continued to be "involved in the evil" of "conjuring," and he attempted to stamp out such activities. Butrick recorded, "I told the congregation that my object was not to please or displease but simply to make known in the clearest manner possible the duty of praying to God alone, & the great evil & wickedness of addressing our prayers to inferior objects." He added that as "I had the whole system of conjuration in my mind I endeavored to expose its weakness, folly & guilt as far as possible." Charles Moore took great exception and stormed out of the service. Afterward he approached the minister and forced him to look at his ill son. Sores covered the poor boy's arm, and Moore stated that "those may be there till he dies" without the attention of a practitioner. "At this the whole church forsook me," Butrick reported, "so that the next Sabbath scarcely a Cherokee attended meeting." Attendance of Sunday services continued to drop off thereafter as Hightower's residents "still adhering to their conjuring practices forsook our meetings altogether."[116] For Butrick, true Christians were to look upon the Bible "as not only their food, their medicine, & support but as their light—their guide, their directory, given from heaven."[117] Most Cherokees saw in their practitioners another directory when it came to healing and preventing diseases.

Conclusion

In the fall of 1824, Cherokee leaders authorized a census of their people. The smallpox scare had passed and agents employed by the National Council ventured out into every district and counted how many people resided within their national bounds. Not since 1721, when the British came up with a total of 10,379 Cherokee men, women, and children, had a census with as much exactness been undertaken. When returns rolled in and numbers were added together, the nation counted a total of 13,783 Native citizens, a category that excluded intermarried Euro-Americans and enslaved African Americans.[1] A comparison between the two detailed censuses thus reveals something rather remarkable: the population of an indigenous nation actually increased over a roughly one-hundred-year period in which smallpox threatened every generation. *Variola* circulated near southern Appalachia in 1738, 1749, 1759, 1780, 1806, and 1824, and on each occasion infected at least some Cherokee families and on two occasions—1738–39 and 1759–60—infiltrated a wide proportion of their towns and caused major epidemics. Yet, the Cherokees counted 3,404 more members of their nation in 1824 than the British did in 1721. The difference was even greater as the 1824 census did not include some 500 Cherokees, who at the time of the counting lived on a reservation in North Carolina, and another approximately 3,000, who had by then relocated to the West. If these are added, the total number becomes 17,283, which means there were 6,904 or about 67 percent more Cherokees in 1824 than there had been in 1721.[2]

Can we now conclude that Cherokees were successful in their fight against smallpox? That of course depends on how one defines success. If success is measured in numbers—those that show a Native group's population returning to the level it had been before small-pox arrived, then more questions arise than are answered. First, when did smallpox first arrive? In the case of the Cherokees and so many other indigenous groups, one cannot say definitely when *Variola* first reached them. The preponderance of the evidence indicates that the germ most likely infected Cherokees for the first time around 1698, but an earlier or later initial experience cannot be ruled out. Second, even if one could pinpoint the arrival of smallpox with certainty, how many people did the group have at the time? Determining this is exceedingly difficult, if not impossible. If 1698 marks the begin-ning of the Cherokees' experience with smallpox, one might derive a pre-epidemic number by extrapolating backward from the 1721 census based on several assumptions: What percentage became infected, how many perished, and what was the net change between 1698 and 1721 based on births, deaths, adoption of outsiders, and loss of captives? In chapter 1, the hypothetical example of universal infection, 40 percent mortality rate, and zero population growth was used to derive a pre-epidemic population of 17,298. While this figure is remarkably close to the 17,283 Cherokees in 1824, it is still based on variables that could be changed to produce either a higher or lower pre-1698 population level. Third, the 1721 census should be read critically. The British may have undercounted Cherokees. Presum-ably knowledgeable traders did the counting, but did they count everybody? The British listed a total of fifty-three villages, while traders had noted that at some point the Cherokees had sixty-four villages.[3] Did nine villages go uncounted or were these villages abandoned within the last couple of decades because of population losses from the smallpox epidemic, warfare, or other factors? Perhaps more research will help answer some of these questions, but for now the numbers leave one unsatisfied in interpreting the indigenous experience with colonialism's most dreaded germ.

The theoretical construct of the "virgin soil" thesis should also leave one unsatisfied. First, those who employ this theory often do so with misleading metaphoric language ("seven-league boots," "shock troops")

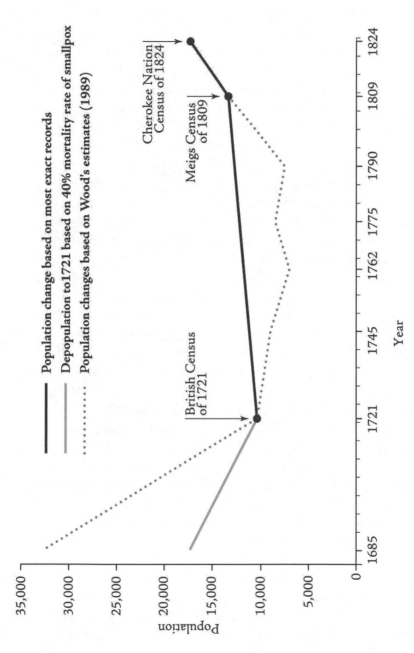

Cherokee population estimates and counts, 1685–1824. Several problematic assumptions lay behind the choices of where to peg Cherokee population before smallpox arrived. One choice makes their more certain number in 1824 appear still to be far away from what they once had, while another choice shows a population rebound to what it had been before smallpox arrived. However one reads the "data," smallpox in itself did not result in a linear and irreversible population decline. Populations rebounded after epidemics, only to be cut into by subsequent episodes of colonial violence.

and similes ("spread like wildfire," "radiated like ink"). These obscure the human agency of colonizers that provided the context in which an acute infectious disease spread great distances and produced catastrophic mortality rates. This agency needed not involve the purposeful dissemination of *Variola* through virus-laden blankets and other materials but involved more complicated activities such as the Native slave trade, warfare, sustained commercial intercourse, and scorched-earth military tactics. These provided the conditions for *Variola* to reach southern Appalachia, to spread from village to village after it arrived, and to exact high casualty rates. Second, the theory denigrates indigenous peoples as passive victims who had no agency of their own in combating the virus. The Cherokees' experience demonstrates the fallaciousness of this presumed impotence. Their practitioners responded actively and did so with some effectiveness: they incorporated smallpox into their cosmology, constructed rituals to deal with the contagious pathogen, advised their followers to avoid exposure, and secluded those who became infected. Such efforts were not always successful as demonstrated by the 1759–60 epidemic, an event necessarily linked to the larger Anglo-British War prosecuted so ruthlessly by Sir Jeffery Amherst. Third, the "virgin soil" thesis overwhelmingly relies on anecdotal type of evidence that, when subject to critical analysis, does not always bear up as factual. James Adair's infamous account of the 1738–39 epidemic clearly has fundamental problems including an exaggeration of the outbreak's impact and mischaracterization of Native responses. John Carr's memory of smallpox exacting retribution on the Cherokees for murdering settlers in 1780—a memory formulated in part from a reading of Adair's previous account—presents a more egregious case in which scholars have been misled into believing a catastrophic epidemic occurred when no corroborating evidence that dates to the revolution confirms such an event.

Finally, the "virgin soil" thesis creates a deterministic narrative of inevitable declension of Native peoples both in terms of their numbers and their culture. Cherokee numbers again remain problematic, but there are reasons to believe that following their initial experience with smallpox that their population would have thereafter increased and eventually reached its pre-epidemic level within a few generations, if nondisease factors of colonialism had not interfered. Cherokees in other words suffered a series of traumas that cut into population gains they made after previous epidemics. Had the Anglo-Cherokee War and the American Revolution not intervened, Cherokees would have reached the seventeen thousand mark much sooner than 1824. Vaccination certainly helped protect Cherokees from smallpox-induced mortality, but even before this procedure became widely accepted in their nation, they had substantially rebuilt their population. Vaccine in other words was only one factor and not the most important one in the resurgence of Cherokee population. That Cherokees accepted this procedure, moreover, does not take away from what their practitioners had accomplished in regard to protecting their people from smallpox and other introduced diseases. Cherokees accepted this vaccine on their own terms and did so without turning their back on their own medical beliefs and practices. Even with the frightening mortality from colonial germs, violent deaths and famines produced by invading armies, derogatory measures taken by missionaries, and the revolutionary breakthrough that vaccine provided in fighting smallpox, Cherokee medicine remained vital to Cherokee people well into the nineteenth century and beyond.

The "virgin soil" thesis thus covers up more than it reveals. This theoretical construct most unfortunately masks Native voices that described what they experienced and how they endured as a people. With research that goes beyond the disparate references produced by colonists over a vast time and space, one can find these hitherto muted voices in the historical record. Meeting with representatives from the state of Virginia at the end of the revolution, for example, a Cherokee delegation sought peace and asked a question—a very important question that turns out to be central to this book. The delegation said, "Look back and recollect what a numerous and warlike people we were, when our assistance were asked against the French on the Ohio—we took pity on you then, and assisted you. We have been continually since, decreasing, and are now become weak. What are the causes?" Modern students and scholars of history would all do well to listen to their answer: "War, and succeeding invasions of our Country."[4] One year later, Savanukeh echoed his countrymen's conclusions. He journeyed to Saint Augustine, Florida, to plead with the British not to abandon them to the vengeful Americans, exclaiming to Colonel Thomas Brown: "As men and warriors we faced the enemy many of our people fell and our corn was thrice destroyed. . . . We subsisted our women and children on acorns & by hunting and were determined to hold the English fast by the arm and like men stand or fall with our friends." He could not believe, however, that the British had agreed to a peace that left Cherokee lands in American possession. He remarked in dismay, "We have heard from the Virginians that the English have smoked the pipe of peace with their enemies and have given up our lands and yours to be divided amongst their enemies. The peacemakers and our enemies have talked away our lands at a rum drinking."[5] Savanukeh said nothing of smallpox or any other disease. Instead, he stated what the historical record makes clear: American armies and their scorched-earth tactics proved most destructive to the health and well-being of Cherokees during the American Revolution, and in the end human agents and not their supposed biological allies forcefully dispossessed his people of their land.

Tragically, Savanukeh's descendants would again experience another violent form of colonialism in the 1830s. Then, the United States enacted its removal policy and forced nearly the entire Cherokee Nation to relocate to the West. Scholars widely believe that over four thousand, or about one-quarter of the indigenous nation, perished as result of this policy. A population that had recovered from colonialism's past traumas—perhaps even to the degree that it surpassed its pre-1698 level—suffered a major setback again.[6] Deaths occurred as they usually do in such situations of intense colonial violence: diseases—particularly whooping cough, measles, influenza, and cholera (all of which had been introduced after 1492)—combined with malnutrition, exposure, and psychological trauma to produce shocking mortality both in the concentration camps in which Cherokees were collected before their forced march and on their Trail of Tears to what now is the state of Oklahoma.[7] These deaths were certainly not the result of the independent actions of colonial germs. Cherokees never would have been in a situation in which they suffered so severely from diseases without the political decisions made by human actors who put Euro-American desire for Native lands above humane considerations for the lives of indigenous peoples.

Even after this trauma, Cherokee medicine continued to endure and did so in a novel way that began to develop before removal. By the early 1820s, Sequoyah, a Cherokee man known also as George Guess, had invented a way in which his people could communicate in writing in their own language. The alphabet, or more precisely syllabary, that he created had eighty-six characters, each of which represented a distinct syllable of the Cherokee language, and its invention made Sequoyah the only known person in recorded history from a nonliterate nation to have created a system of writing. Seemingly overnight his countrymen became literate in their own language. Rev. William Chamberlain remarked, "A great part of the Cherokees can read and write in their own language. The knowledge of Mr. Guess' alphabet is spreading through the nation like fire among the leaves and it cannot be stopped until the whole nation will be able to read and write."[8] Christians, to be sure, co-opted this syllabary for the purposes of spreading the Gospel. Through their converted interpreters they translated the Bible, hymns, and other Christian materials and disseminated these widely. Practitioners, however, also took up their pens for the promotion of their cosmology. Partly in response to attacks on their beliefs and practices, they recorded their formulas.[9] They exchanged these to other practitioners and to future generations. While practitioners continued to train their apprentices as they had before and passed on knowledge orally, the written formulas became the basis of much of the knowledge that scholars have today of Cherokee medicine. Altogether these formulas provide a rich legacy, one in which human survival depends on collective actions to maintain reciprocal relationships with each other and with multiple spirit beings that inhabit the cosmos.

NOTES

SOURCE ABBREVIATIONS

ABCFM   American Board of Commissioners for Foreign Missions
               Records. Houghton Library, Harvard University, Cambridge,
               Mass., microfilm.

APSS   *Amherst Papers, 1756–1763, The Southern Sector: Dispatches
               from South Carolina, Virginia and His Majesty's Superintendent
               of Indian Affairs*. Edith Mays, ed. Westminster, Md.: Heritage
               Books, 2006.

BJ   *The Brainerd Journal: A Mission to the Cherokees, 1817–1823*.
               Joyce B. Phillips and Paul Gary Phillips, eds. Lincoln: Uni-
               versity of Nebraska Press, 1998.

BLP   Benjamin Lincoln Papers. Massachusetts Historical Society,
               Boston, microfilm.

BPROSC   *Records in the British Public Records Office Relating to South
               Carolina*. Transcribed by W. Noel Sainsbury. 36 vols. South
               Carolina Department of History and Archives, Columbia,
               1955, microfilm.

C.O.   Colonial Office Records. National Archives of the United
               Kingdom (formerly known as the British Public Record Office).
               Transcripts and microfilm at Library of Congress, Washing-
               ton, D.C. and Hunter Library, Western Carolina University,
               Cullowhee, N.C.

CP   *The Cornwallis Papers*. Ian Saberton, ed. 6 vols. East Sussex,
               U.K: Naval and Military Press, 2010.

CRG   *Colonial Records of the State of Georgia*. Allen Candler, Lucian
               Knight, Kenneth Coleman, and Milton Ready, eds. 39 vols.
               Atlanta: Franklin Printing and Publishing; Athens: Univer-
               sity of Georgia Press, 1904–.

CSRNC	*The Colonial and State Records of North Carolina*. William L. Saunders and Walter Clark, eds. 26 vols. Raleigh: P. M. Hale, 1886–1907.
CVSP	*Calendar of Virginia State Papers and Other Manuscripts*. William Palmer et al., eds. 11 vols. Richmond: Virginia State Library, 1875–93.
Draper Mss.	Lyman Copeland Draper Manuscripts. Wisconsin Historical Society, Madison, microfilm.
DRIA, 1	*Documents Relating to Indian Affairs, 1750-1754*. William L. McDowell, Jr., ed. Columbia: South Carolina Archives Department, 1958.
DRIA, 2	*Documents Relating to Indian Affairs, 1754-1765*. William L. McDowell, Jr., ed. Columbia: University of South Carolina Press, 1970.
DSC	*The De Soto Chronicles: The Expedition of Hernando de Soto to the United States, 1539–1543*. Langdon Clayton and Vernon Knight, eds. 2 vols. Tuscaloosa: University of Alabama, 1993.
Forbes Papers	Headquarters Papers of General John Forbes Relating to the Expedition against Fort Duquesne. University of Virginia Library. Charlottesville, microfilm.
Gage Papers	General Thomas Gage. Papers. William L. Clements Library, University of Michigan, Ann Arbor.
Greene Papers	*The Papers of General Nathanael Greene*. Richard Showman, ed. 13 vols. Chapel Hill: University of North Carolina Press, 1976–2005.
Haldimand Papers	Sir Frederick Haldimand. Unpublished Papers and Correspondence, 1758–84. British Museum, London, microfilm.
HQP	British Headquarters (Sir Guy Carleton) Papers. Colonial Williamsburg Foundation, microfilm.
JCHASC	*The Journal of the Commons House of Assembly of South Carolina*. Alexander S. Salley, ed. 21 vols. Columbia: South Carolina Department of Archives and History, 1907–49.
JCHASC	The Journal of the Commons House of Assembly of South Carolina. Transcripts. South Carolina Department of Archives and History, microfilm.
JCIT	*Journals of the Commissioners of the Indian Trade, September 20, 1710–August 29, 1718*. William L. McDowell, ed. Columbia: South Carolina Archives Department, 1955.
JPE	*The Juan Pardo Expeditions: Exploration of the Carolinas and Tennessee, 1566–1568*. Charles Hudson, ed., with documents relating to the Pardo Expedition transcribed, translated, and annotated by Paul E. Hoffman. Washington, D.C.: Smithsonian Institution Press, 1990.

LOC	Library of Congress, Washington, D.C.
M15	Secretary of War. Letters Sent Relating to Indian Affairs, 1800–1824. National Archives and Records Administration, Washington, D.C., microfilm.
M208	Records of the Cherokee Agency in Tennessee. National Archives and Records Administration, Washington, D.C., microfilm.
M234	Office of Indians Affairs. Letters Received, 1824–81. National Archives and Records Administration, Washington, D.C., microfilm.
MAB	Moravian Mission Records. Moravian Archives. Bethlehem, Pa., microfilm.
MAS	Letters. Moravian Archives. Salem, N.C.
MSMC	*The Moravian Springplace Mission to the Cherokees.* Rowena McClinton, ed. 2 vols. Lincoln: University of Nebraska Press, 2007.
MPAFD	*Mississippi Provincial Archives, French Dominion.* Dunbar Rowland, A. G. Sanders, and Patricia Galloway, eds. 5 vols. Jackson: Mississippi Department of Archives and History, 1927–32 and 1984.
NARA	National Archives and Records Administration, Washington, D.C.
NYCD	*Documents Relative to the Colonial History of the State of New York.* Edmund O'Callaghan, John Brodhead, and Berthold Fernow, eds. 15 vols. Albany: Weed, Parsons, and Company, 1853–87.
NYPL	New York Public Library, New York.
Payne-Butrick	*The Payne-Butrick Papers.* William L. Anderson, Anne F. Rogers, and Jane L. Brown, eds. 2 vols. Lincoln: University of Nebraska Press, 2010.
PTJ	*Papers of Thomas Jefferson.* Julian P. Bond et al., eds. 39 vols. Princeton, N.J.: Princeton University Press, 1950–.
RG	Record Group.
RSUS	Records of the States of the United States of America. Library of Congress, Washington, D.C., microfilm.
RWP	Revolutionary War Pension and Bounty—Land Warrant Application Files. National Archives and Records Administration. Washington, D.C. Digital Copies through Fold3. http://www.fold3.com/.
SPG	Records of the Society for the Propagation of the Gospel. Society for the Propagation of the Gospel in Foreign Parts. London, microfilm.
SWJP	*The Papers of Sir William Johnson.* James Sullivan et al., eds. 14 vols. Albany: University of the State of New York, 1921–65.

WHL   William Henry Lyttelton. Papers. William L. Clements Library,
                             University of Michigan, Ann Arbor.
W.O.   War Office Records. National Archives of the United King-
                             dom (formerly known as the British Public Record Office).
                             Transcripts and microfilm at Library of Congress, Washing-
                             ton, D.C.

Introduction

1. Heckewelder, *A Narrative of the Mission of the United Brethren*, 200–202. Heckewelder refers to Savanukeh as "the Crow," but American and British records at
the time most often call him "the Raven." English speakers also used the name
"Delawares" when referring to the Lenapes. Here and throughout this book spelling, capitalization, and punctuation in the original quotes have been corrected and
standardized when appropriate to accord with modern conventions for the conve-
nience of the reader. The intrusive insertion of *sic* will not be employed. Insertions
by the author will be indicated by the use of brackets and deletions will be indicated by ellipses.

2. Broadhead to the Delawares, June 22, 1779, in Kellogg, ed., *Frontier Advance*, 368.

3. "Recollections of Stephen Burkam" in ibid., 157.

4. Heckewelder, *Narrative*, 192–93. Heckewelder mistakenly gives the year of
White Eye's death as 1780 in his recollection.

5. Morgan to the President of Congress, May 12, 1784, Papers of the Continental Congress, NARA, RG 360, M247, item 163, roll 180, pp. 365–67, http://www.
fold3.com/image/393887/ (accessed May 30, 2013).

6. On smallpox during the revolution, see Fenn, *Pox Americana*.

7. Francisco de Aguilar, "Eighth Jornada," in Schwartz, ed., *Victors and Vanquished*, 198.

8. Winthrop to D'Ewes, July 21, 1634, in *Winthrop Papers*, 3:171–72.

9. Archdale, "A New Description of that Fertile and Pleasant Province of Carolina," in Salley, ed., *Narratives of Early Carolina*, 285.

10. For other examples of European interpretations of these events, see Jones,
Rationalizing Epidemics, 21–67.

11. Crosby, "Virgin Soil Epidemics," 289–99, quotes on 289 and 290.

12. Ibid., 296.

13. Crosby, *Ecological Imperialism*, 196.

14. Dobyns, *Their Number Become Thinned*, 8.

15. Dobyns, "Estimating Aboriginal American Population," 395–416. Dobyns's
methods and conclusions have been subjected to much criticism yet he maintained
his stance for the remainder of his career. The most critical assessment is Henige,
Numbers from Nowhere. For a summary of the debate as it pertains to North America,
see Daniels, "The Indian Population of North America in 1492." This study continues

the critical view of Dobyns's suggestions of early hemispheric pandemics that scholars in the 1980s initiated. See also Milner, "Epidemic Disease in the Postcontact Southeast"; Snow and Lanphear, "European Contact and Indian Depopulation in the Northeast"; Reff, *Disease, Depopulation, and Culture Change*; Warrick, "European Infectious Disease and Depopulation of the Wendat-Tionontate." By doubting early pandemics, these works challenge the high estimates of aboriginal population that Dobyns proposed but nonetheless do not question other aspects of the "virgin soil" thesis.

16. Diamond, *Guns, Germs, and Steel*, 373–74.

17. Mann, *1491*, 61.

18. Ibid., 93.

19. Talk of Cherokee Nation delivered by the Raven of Chottee at Savannah, September 1, 1781, C.O., 5/82/287.

20. The supposed epidemic of 1780 and the historians who have cited its occurrence as an actual fact will be discussed in chapter 4.

21. Other works have offered critiques of particular aspects of the "virgin soil" thesis and my work is indebted to this body of scholarship. Fenn does not make an explicit critique of the "virgin soil" thesis in either *Pox Americana* or "Biological Warfare in Eighteenth Century North America." But, she nonetheless puts the spread of smallpox into the context of the upheavals of the American Revolution in her book and suggests in her article that deliberate attempts to infect Native Americans likely occurred more often than the one documented account at Fort Pitt in 1763. Jones has offered the most cogent challenge to Crosby's conclusions and points to a number of studies who carelessly read Crosby to mean Natives had deficient genes. There is no evidence for this genetic weakness as will be discussed later in this introduction. Jones concludes that factors other than lack of acquired immunity and genetics—such as poverty, inequality, and exploitation—must be considered for the deleterious health consequences that indigenous peoples faced. See Jones, "Virgin Soils Revisited," and Jones, *Rationalizing Epidemics*. Alchon, Bacci, Kelm, and Lux also have moved us away from a singular focus on infectious diseases and highlight the multiple causes of Native health disparities and depopulation. See Alchon, *A Pest in the Land*; Bacci, *Conquest*; Kelm, *Colonizing Bodies*; and Lux, *Medicine that Walks*. I made a similar argument in *Epidemics and Enslavement*. These studies move us into a fruitful direction by illustrating how the nondisease factors of colonialism are more important considerations in assessing depopulation because they interfered with Native fertility and recovery from disease-induced depopulation. The studies cited above also serve as a starting point in assessing how indigenous peoples exercised their own agency in attempting to protect themselves, and yet how colonialism interfered with those attempts. I summarily developed this idea in an earlier work and will expand and refine it in chapter 2 of this book. See Kelton, "Avoiding the Smallpox Spirits: Colonial Epidemics and Southeastern Indian Survival," *Ethnohistory* 51 (Winter 2004): 45–71. For a more thorough review of the literature on the topic, see Jones, "Death, Uncertainty, and Rhetoric," in Cameron, Kelton, and Swedlund, eds., *Beyond Germs*.

22. Adair, *History of the American Indians*, 252.

23. Ibid., 252–53.

24. The literature on the Cherokees during the time period that this book covers is vast, certainly in large part because of the large number of sources and prominent role the indigenous nation played in historical developments. This work is indebted to the following insightful and relatively recent studies: McLoughlin, *Cherokee Renascence*; Hatley, *Dividing Paths*; Hoig, *The Cherokees and Their Chiefs*; Perdue, *Cherokee Women*; Oliphant, *Peace and War on the Anglo-Cherokee Frontier*; Cumfer, *Separate Peoples, One Land*; Miles, *The House on Diamond Hill*; Boulware, *Deconstructing the Cherokee Nation*. The demographic works of Thornton and Wood include the Cherokees' experience with smallpox and inform this study. See Thornton, *The Cherokees*; Wood, "The Impact of Smallpox on the Native Population of the 18th-century South," and "The Changing Population of the Colonial South."

25. Chin, ed., *Control of Communicable Diseases Manual*, 455–57; Shurkin, *Invisible Fire*, 26–27. A milder strain of smallpox, *Variola minor*, has been identified, but the more severe form, *Variola major*, appeared predominately during the colonial era.

26. Chin, *Control of Communicable Diseases Manual*, 455–57; Shurkin, *Invisible Fire*, 26–27.

27. Chin, *Control of Communicable Diseases Manual*, 270–76.

28. Ibid., 330–35.

29. Chin, *Control of Communicable Diseases Manual*, 553–58; Ackerknect, *History and Geography of the Most Important Diseases*, 34–35; Cooper and Kiple, "Yellow Fever," 1100–1107.

30. Chin, *Control of Communicable Diseases Manual*, 381–87; McNeil, *Plagues and Peoples*, 161–207.

31. Chin, *Control of Communicable Diseases Manual*, 541–44; Ackerknect, *History and Geography of the Most Important Diseases*, 34–35; Zinsser, *Rats, Lice, and History*.

32. Ramenofsky, "Diseases of the Americas, 1492–1700."

33. Chin, *Control of Communicable Diseases Manual*, 535–41; LeBaron and Taylor, "Typhoid Fever," 1071–77.

34. Merbs, "New World of Infectious Disease."

35. Chin, *Control of Communicable Diseases Manual*, 381–87; Harder, "The Seeds of Malaria."

36. Jones identifies several particular incidences of this misinterpretation in "Virgin Soils Revisited."

37. Barquet and Domingo, "Smallpox." This and the nine previous paragraphs summarize a more lengthy discussion that can be found in Kelton, *Epidemics and Enslavement*, 44–45, where I discuss the possibility of genetic homogeneity as playing a role in driving up mortality rates. Because RNA-virus can rapidly alter their genetic structures in response to the human immune system, they become more virulent when passed from one individual to a genetically similar individual such as a sibling. Some scientists speculate that indigenous communities being comparatively small in scale and isolated must have had a high degree of genetic homogeneity

and thus were susceptible to higher mortality. Other scholars are not convinced about the degree of genetic homogeneity. In any event, I did not emphasize in my earlier work that smallpox is a DNA-virus. These viruses, as James Riley discusses, are "comparatively stable" unlike RNA-viruses such as influenza, mumps, measles, and the common cold. Genetic homogeneity, if it indeed characterized most indigenous communities, thus cannot be considered as a major factor in driving up mortality rates from smallpox. See Riley, "Smallpox and American Indians Revisited," 468.

CHAPTER 1

1. Dobyns, *Their Number Become Thinned*, 11.

2. Crosby, "Virgin Soil Epidemics," 290.

3. Crosby, *Ecological Imperialism*, 201.

4. Mann, *1491*, 87.

5. Axtell, *Natives and Newcomers*, 44–45.

6. Kennedy et al., *The American Pageant*, 15. A more nuanced argument for early, undocumented epidemics is Ramenofsky, *Vectors of Death*.

7. Kelton, *Epidemics and Enslavement*, 146–47 and162; *JCIT*, 266 and 272–73.

8. Snow and Lanphear, "European Contact and Indian Depopulation in the Northeast," 23.

9. Worth, *The Timucuan Chiefdoms*, 2:10; Hann, *Apalachee*, 176–77.

10. Dobyns, *Their Number Become Thinned*, 12–13; Cook, *Born to Die*, 60–85.

11. "A True & Exact account of the number & names of all the Towns belonging to the Cherrikeee Nation & the Number of Men, Women & Children Inhabiting the Same taken Anno 1721," SPG, ser. A, vol. 18: 75–76.

12. Townsend, *The Aztecs*, 82–93.

13. Livi Bacci, *Conquest*, 53–55; Cook, *Born to Die*, 70–72; Alchon, *Pest in the Land*, 64–67.

14. Cook, *Born to Die*, 72–85; Alchon, *Pest in the Land*, 66–68 and 75. Livi Bacci dissents from this conclusion, see *Conquest*, 55–56 and 61.

15. Reff, *Disease, Depopulation, Culture Change*, 102–103.

16. The literature on chiefdoms in the Southeast is vast. A particular good summary is Widmer, "The Structure of Southeastern Chiefdoms," 125–55.

17. Hally, "Chiefdom of Coosa," 227–53.

18. On Cahokia, see Pauketat, *Ascent of Chiefs*; Pauketat and Emerson, *Cahokia*; Emerson, *Cahokia and the Archaeology of Power*. On Cahokia being exceptional, see Muller, *Mississippian Political Economy*.

19. On Cherokee settlement and subsistence patterns, see Ward and Davis, *Time before History*, 160–61; Dickens, "Mississippian Settlement Patterns in the Appalachian Summit Area," 115–39; Dickens, *Cherokee Prehistory*, 46–51. On economic redundancy and self-sufficiency of southeastern chiefdoms, see Blitz, *Ancient Chiefdoms of the Tombigbee*, 105; Muller, *Mississippian Political Economy*, 252.

20. For incoming items, see Roberts, "Lythic Artifacts," 822–24; Peebles and Kus, "Some Archaeological Correlates of Ranked Societies," 443; Steponaitis, "Contrasting Patterns of Mississippian Development," 208–16. For outgoing items, see Dickens, *Cherokee Prehistory*, 156–58.

21. Hally, "The Chiefdom of Coosa," 243.

22. Welch, *Moundville's Economy*, 194–97.

23. Milner, Anderson, and Smith, "Distribution of Eastern Woodlands Peoples," 16; Griffin, "Comments on Late Prehistoric Societies," 10–11.

24. Larson, "Functional Considerations of Warfare in the Southeast," 383–392; Gibson, "Aboriginal Warfare in the Protohistoric Southeast," 130–33; Dickson, "Yanomamö of the Mississippi Valley," 909–16; Steinen, "Ambushes, Raids, and Palisades," 132–39.

25. Hickerson, *The Southwestern Chippewa*, 12–29.

26. Anderson, "Stability and Change," 208.

27. Hudson, *Knights of Spain*, 209.

28. Dickens, "Mississippian Settlement Patterns in the Appalachian Summit," 115–39; Ward and Davis, *Time before History*, 160–61.

29. For appraisals of long-distance trade during the precontact period, see Peebles and Kus, "Some Archaeological Correlates of Ranked Societies," 443; Steponaitis, "Contrasting Patterns of Mississippian Development," 208–16. I have critiqued the idea of smallpox's spread into the Mississippi Valley in the 1520s in more detail elsewhere; see Kelton, *Epidemics and Enslavement*, 38–42 and 48–50.

30. Axtell, *Natives and Newcomers*, 230–31; Crosby, *Ecological Imperialism*, 213–14; Diamond, *Guns, Germs, Steel*, 211 and 373–74; Dobyns, *Their Number Become Thinned*, 250–74; Ramenofsky and Galloway, "Disease and the Soto Entrada," 259–80, especially 274.

31. Kelton, *Epidemics and Enslavement*, 50–82.

32. "The Account by a Gentleman from Elvas," in *DSC*, 1: 83.

33. Garcilaso de la Vega, "La Florida by the Inca," in *DSC*, 2:286.

34. "The Account by a Gentleman from Elvas," in *DSC*, 1: 84; Biedma, "Relation of the Island of Florida," in *DSC*, 1:231.

35. Widmer, "The Structure of Southeastern Chiefdoms," 137–38; Chester DePratter, "The Chiefdom of Cofitachequi," 215–16.

36. Hudson and his associates have done excellent work recalibrating Soto's and Pardo's paths to a more northward passage across the Appalachians whereas earlier scholars believed the passage occurred either through the location where the Cherokees existed in the eighteenth century or to the south. See Hudson, *The Juan Pardo Expeditions*, and Hudson, *Knights of Spain*. Further archaeological investigation has modified Hudson's reconstruction but keeps the route to the north. My study utilizes the routes sketched out in Beck, "From Joara to Chiaha," 162–69.

37. Hudson, *Knights of Spain*, 185–219.

38. "Account by a Gentleman from Elvas," in *DSC*, 1:86; "Account by Rangel," in *DSC*, 1:281.

39. Hudson, *Knights of Spain*, 186.

40. Moore, *Catawba Valley Mississippian*, 188, 190, 191, and 194; Hudson, *Knights of Spain*, 187.

41. "Account by a Gentleman from Elvas," in *DSC*, 1:87; "Short Bandera Relation," in *JPE*, 302–303; and "Long Bandera Account," in *JPE*, 277–78. (Joara appears as "Xuala" in *The De Soto Chronicles*.) For location of these towns, see Beck, "From Joara to Chiaha," 162–69. On cultural identification of Joara, see Beck and Moore, "The Burke Phase," 194 and 201. Two other towns on the Nolichucky that Pardo entered, Guasili and Canasagua, appear to be Cherokee in origin but do not have a clear equivalent on later town lists. Canasagua, however, was a common place name among the Cherokees who called a creek that flowed into the Hiwassee River, "Ganasa'gi." See Goodwin, *Cherokees in Transition*, 153–54.

42. Goodwin, *Cherokees in Transition*, 153–56.

43. Beck, "From Joara to Chiaha," 167.

44. "Long Bandera Account," in *JPE*, 266–67.

45. Goodwin, *Cherokees in Transition*, 153–56; Hudson, *Knights of Spain*, 193 and 199.

46. Beck and Moore identify Chisca with the Saltville archaeological site in the forks of the Holston but have not concluded that it is directly ancestral to the Cherokees. See Beck and Moore, "The Burke Phase," 192. On chiefdom development in southwestern Virginia, see Meyers, "The Mississippian Frontier in Southwestern Virginia," 178–91.

47. Mooney, *History, Myths*, 380–81.

48. Henderson, "Treaty of Long Island of the Holston, July 1777," 83; Mooney, *History, Myths*, 341–42 and 388–89; and Hicks to Ross, February 1, 1826, in Moulton, ed., *Papers of Chief John Ross*, 1:112.

49. Norton, *Journal*, 44.

50. Hicks to Ross, February 1, 1826, in Moulton, *Papers of Chief John Ross*, 1:112.

51. "Cherokee Traditions." One last bit of evidence that suggests a connection is the name Chisca itself. It may be the Cherokee word for bird, "Jiskwa." Of course, Chisca could have been a name applied to a people rather than one that they called themselves; the Spanish learned the name from the Chisca's enemies, and it could have also been a mere coincidence that the name sounds like the Cherokee word for bird.

52. Smith, *Archaeology of Aboriginal Culture Change*, 137–38

53. Chapman, *Tellico Archaeology*, 99–100; Smith, *Coosa*, 96–117.

54. Norton, *Journal*, 108.

55. Hudson, *Knights of Spain*, 73–74.

56. "Account of Biedma," in *DSC*, 1:231; "Account by a Gentleman from Elvas," in *DSC*, 1:87.

57. "Account by a Gentleman from Elvas," in *DSC*, 1:89.

58. Ibid., 1:91.

59. "Account of Rodrigo Rangel," in *DSC*, 1:285.

60. "Account by a Gentleman from Elvas," in *DSC*, 1:93.

61. "Martinez Relation," in *JPE*, 320. Later accounts suggest that Joara's warriors were enemies to Chisca and went along with Moyano. See *JPE*, 27–28.

62. Meyers, "Mississippian Frontier in Southwestern Virginia," 178–91.

63. Thanks to the remarkable work of an archaeological team led by Robin Beck, Jr., the site where Fort San Juan stood has been identified and excavated. See Beck et al, "Identifying Fort San Juan," 65–77. For a more in-depth look at relations between Pardo's men and indigenous peoples, see Beck et al, "Limiting Resistance," 19–39. For a larger perspective on violence between Spanish explorers and indigenous peoples, see Beck et al, "Conflict Violence, and Warfare in *La Florida*," 232–49.

64. Quoted in Worth, *Timucuan Chiefdoms*, 2:10–11.

65. Hann, *Apalachee*, 176–77; and Hann, "Translation of Governor Robolledo's 1657 Visitation," 109.

66. Worth, *Timucuan Chiefdom*, 2:10.

67. Hann, "Translation of Governor Robolledo's 1657 Visitation," 92.

68. Waselkov, "Macon Trading House," 194; and Waselkov, "Seventeenth-Century Trade in the Colonial Southeast," 117–33.

69. Schlesier, "Epidemics and Indian Middlemen," 129–45; Richter, *Ordeal of the Longhouse*, 145.

70. Robinson, "An Indian King's Will," 192–93.

71. Blanton, *Medicine in Virginia in the Seventeenth Century*, 60–61.

72. Aquila, *The Iroquois Restoration*, 205–10.

73. Various perspectives on the Native slave trade can be found in Ethridge and Shuck-Hall, eds., *Mapping the Mississippian Shatter Zone*. See also Gallay, *The Indian Slave Trade*; Oatis, *A Colonial Complex*. Colonialism created shatter zones throughout the Americas. For a particularly insightful analysis of this phenomenon, see Blackhawk, *Violence over the Land*.

74. Perdue, *Cherokee Women*, 53–55.

75. Kelton, *Epidemics and Enslavement*, 129, 136, 140, and 149.

76. White, *The Roots of Dependency*, 58–59. For an overview of Natives and alcohol during the colonial era, see Mancall, *Deadly Medicine*. For a more comprehensive view of the Cherokees' attempts to deal with alcohol, see Ishii, *Bad Fruits of the Civilized Tree*.

77. Bowne, *The Westo Indians*.

78. Merrell, *The Indians' New World*, 27–48.

79. Mooney, *History, Myths*, 381.

80. "Letter of Abraham Wood Describing Needham's Journey (1673)," in Williams, ed., *Early Travels in the Tennessee Country*, 17–38.

81. Chicken, "A Journal from Carolina in 1715 [1716]," 330. Discourse between Long Warrior of Tunnisee, head warrior and president of South Carolina Council, January 24, 1727, C.O., 5/387/237.

82. Adair, *History of the American Indians*, 273. The ethnic identity and fate of the Tomahitans remains a puzzle. Swanton suggested that they were Yuchi and became incorporated into the Creek Confederacy. (See Swanton, *Early History of the Creek*

Indians, 184–91.) Bowne suggests that they were Cherokees but does not speculate on their ultimate fate. (See Bowne, *The Westo Indians*, 13, 30–31, 33.)

83. On Bacon's Rebellion, see Schmidt, *The Divided Dominion*.

84. Byrd, *Writings*, 185.

85. Alvord and Bidgood, *First Explorations of the Trans-Allegheny Region*, 31.

86. "1681 Census of Guale and Mocama," in Worth, ed., *Struggle for the Georgia Coast*, 101.

87. Boyd, ed., "Expedition of Marcus Delgado," 26. Boyd, following Delgado's manuscript, gave the spelling of this group as "Qusate."

88. Woodward, "Faithfull Relation of my Westoe Voiage," in Salley, ed., *Narratives of Early Carolina*, 134.

89. Crane, *The Southern Frontier*, 40.

90. Lords Proprietors to Seth Sothell et al., May 13, 1691, *BPROSC*, 2:14–15.

91. Salley, ed., *Journal of the Commons House of Assembly of South Carolina for 1693*, 12.

92. I keep with the pre-1783 spelling "Charles Town." In 1783, the city officially became known as it is now "Charleston."

93. Hewatt, *An Historical Account*, 1:116.

94. I have coined the term "the Great Southeastern Smallpox Epidemic" and discuss it in more detail elsewhere. See Kelton, "The Great Southeastern Smallpox Epidemic" in Ethridge and Hudson, eds., *The Transformation of the Southeastern Indians*, 21–37; and Kelton, *Epidemics and Enslavement*, 143–58.

95. Traunter, "Travels between Virginian and South Carolina, 1698–99."

96. Blake and Council to the Proprietors, April 23, 1698, in Salley, ed., *Commissions and Instructions from the Lords Proprietors*, 105.

97. Coming to Sister, March 6, 1699 quoted in McCrady, *History of South Carolina*, 1:308.

98. Pénicaut, *Fleur de Lys and Calumet*, 11.

99. Le Moyne d'Iberville, *Gulf Journals*, 38; Pénicaut, *Fleur de Lys and Calumet*, 11.

100. Le Moyne d'Iberville, *Gulf Journals*, 63.

101. "Letter of J. F. Buisson St. Cosme," in Shea, ed., *Early Voyages up and down the Mississippi*, 72–73.

102. Scholars often state as a matter of fact that smallpox struck Cherokees in 1697 or 1698 but the trail of citations does not lead back to actual documentary evidence that identifies Cherokees as victims of the disease. Hatley, *The Dividing Paths*, 6; Wood, "The Changing Population of the Colonial South," 63; Reid, *A Better Kind of Hatchet*, 30; Crane, *Southern Frontier*, 142.

103. Adair, *History of the American Indians*, 252.

104. Thomas Eyre to Robert Eyre, December 4, 1740, in Lane, ed., *General Oglethorpe's Georgia*, 2:505–507.

105. Moore to [Trustees], September 14, 1739, *CRG*, 5:229; Oglethorpe to Verelst, October 19, 1739, *CRG*, 22 (part 2):244–49.

106. "A True & Exact account of the Number of Names of all the Towns belonging to the Cherrikee Nation & the Number of Men Women & Children Inhabiting the same taken Anno 1721," SPG, Ser. A, 17:155–58.

107. Bull to Lords Commissioners of Trade and Plantations, June 15, 1742, *BPROSC*, 20:568.

108. Hicks to Ross, May 4, 1826, Moulton, *Papers of Chief John Ross*, 1:117.

109. Memorial of Robert Bunning and Others, November 22, 1751, *DRIA*, 1:148.

110. Moore, ed., *Nairne's Muskhogean Journals*, 76.

111. Reid, *A Better Kind of Hatchet*, 36–38.

112. On the Tuscarora War, see La Vere, *The Tuscarora War*.

113. JCHASC microfilm, May 15, 1711, p. 303 and 333; October 26, 1711, p. 341; Dennis to the Secretary, October 7, 1711, SPG, Ser. A, vol. 6, reel 3; Spotswood to Lord Dartmouth, December 28, 1711, Brock, ed., *Official Letters of Spotswood*, 1:134–38; Commissary Johnston's Notitia Parochialis, 1711–1712, SPG, Ser. A, vol. 7, reel 3.

114. Johnston to Secretary, November 16, 1711, Klingberg, ed., *Papers of Gideon Johnston*, 99.

115. I emphasize demographic collapse as leading to the Yamasee War in "Shattered and Infected: Epidemics and the Origins of the Yamasee War, 1696–1715," in Ethridge and Shuck-Hall, eds., *Mapping the Mississippian Shatter Zone*, 312–32. For other interpretations of the war's causes, see William L. Ramsey, "'Something Cloudy in Their Looks,'" 44–75; Richard L. Haan, "'The Trade Do's Not Flourish as Formerly,'" 341–58; Oatis, *A Colonial Complex*, 113–39; Hahn, *Invention of the Creek Nation*, 74–80.

116. Chicken, "A Journal from Carolina in 1715 [1716]," 330; Discourse between Long Warrior of Tunnisee, head warrior and president of South Carolina Council, January 24, 1727, C.O., 5/387/237–38.

117. Gallay, *Indian Slave Trade*, 220; *JCIT*, 49.

118. Chicken, "Journal from Carolina in 1715 [1716]," 334–35.

119. Craven et al. to Lords Commissioners of Trade and Plantations, July 19, 1715, C.O., 5/1265.

120. Le Jau to Secretary, November 28, 1715, in Klingberg, ed., *Carolina Chronicle of Le Jau*, 169.

121. Chicken, "A Journal from Carolina in 1715 [1716]," 331.

122. Ibid., 344.

123. Chicken records a total of twelve Creeks being killed, but other Carolinian sources pushed the number up to nineteen. See Le Jau to Secretary, Marcy 19, 1716 in Klingberg, ed., *Carolina Chronicle of Le Jau*, 175; Commons House of Assembly to Their Agents in Great Britain, March 15, 1716, C.O., 5/1265/48–49.

124. Boone to Lords Commissioners of Trades and Plantations, April 2, 1717, C.O., 5/1265/140.

125. *JCIT*, 266, 272–73; Hassell to Secretary, October 11, 1718, SPG, Ser. A, 13:189–91.

126. *JCIT*, 272–73.

127. Ibid., 311–12.

128. Vassar, ed., "Some Short Remarks on the Indian Trade," 401–23, quotes on 413, 414, 420, and 421.

129. Bienville to Pontchartrain, January 20, 1716, *MPAFD*, 3: 200; Chicken, "A Journal from Carolina in 1715 [1716]," 331.

130. Mooney, *Aboriginal Population of America North of Mexico*, 8; Wood, "Changing Population of the Colonial South," 63.

131. Thornton provides a more in-depth overview of efforts to calculate precontact Cherokee numbers and concludes with the similar degree of uncertainty. See Thornton, *The Cherokees*, 12–18.

CHAPTER 2

1. Crosby, "Virgin Soil Epidemics," 293, 296–98.

2. McNeill, *Plagues and Peoples*, 217.

3. Axtell, *Invasion Within*, 96–97.

4. Reff, *Disease, Depopulation, Culture Change*, xxii, 251, 262–63; Fenn, *Pox Americana*, 142, 258; Watts, *Epidemics and History*, 102–106; Cronon, *Changes in the Land*, 88–89; Calloway, *New Worlds for All*, 25, 33, 38–41, and 71.

5. Martin, *Keepers of the Game*, 53.

6. Ibid., 146. Martin's thesis has caused a great deal of controversy and its applicability or lack of applicability in the case of the Cherokees will be addressed later in this chapter. For critical views of his thesis, see the essays in Krech, ed., *Indians, Animals, and the Fur Trade*.

7. McLoughlin, *Cherokee Renascence in the New Republic*, 17–18.

8. McLoughlin, *Champions of the Cherokees*, 55.

9. Butrick gathered this information for John Howard Payne, who intended to but never did publish a work on Indian antiquities. Butrick's writings, Payne's unpublished manuscript, and other miscellaneous sources are often collectively referred to as the Payne Papers, which are held at the Newberry Library, Chicago. These papers are now published as *The Payne-Butrick Papers* (ed. Anderson, Rogers, and Brown). I utilize Butrick's letters and notes rather than Payne's interpretation of them.

10. The approach I am taking here is called "upstreaming," a common practice within the field of ethnohistory. The approach involves using cultural beliefs and practices found in latter day ethnographic information to understand past actions and events. For an excellent example of the use of this methodology, see Perdue, *Cherokee Women*.

11. Longe, "Small Postscript," 10.

12. Ibid., 20.

13. *Payne-Butrick*, 1:227–28, 231–32, quotes on 231.

14. Ibid., 1:218, 231, 233–34, 244–45, 261; 2:22–23, 35–38.

15. Grant, "Historical Relation of Facts," 57.

16. Cuming, "Journal," 122.

17. For a more thorough discussion of the nature of leadership in the eighteenth century, see Boulware, *Deconstructing the Cherokee Nation*, especially 11–12. Boulware corrects an earlier study by Fred Gearing that suggests a greater bifurcation between war and civil leadership. See Gearing, *Priests and Warriors*.

18. *Payne-Butrick*, 2:32.

19. Norton, *Journal*, 108.

20. *Payne-Butrick*, 1:227, 265, 268–69, 276; 2:81–82.

21. Cuming, "Journal," 123.

22. Richardson Diary, January 14, 1759, NYPL.

23. Demere to Lyttelton, October 26, 1756, *DRIA*, 2:231.

24. Turner to Lyttelton, July 2, 1758, *DRIA*, 2:471.

25. Perdue, *Cherokee Women*, 17–18, 53–56.

26. Cameron to Stuart, October 11, 1773, C.O., 5/75/9.

27. Timberlake, *Memoirs*, 100.

28. Due to their own biases and prejudices, colonial-era and early nineteenth-century Euro-Americans who recorded aspects of this cosmology seldom had the ability, if at all, to discern the deeper meanings of Cherokee stories and practices. For this reason, this section will rely heavily on James Mooney's late nineteenth-century ethnographic works. Mooney, although imperfect, managed to capture much of the deeper meanings of Cherokee stories and practices, and more recent anthropologists have relied on his work to re-create a basic Cherokee cosmology that has persisted within some communities from the precontact period well into the twentieth century. A fine overview of Cherokee cosmology when it comes to medicine that this section extensively draws upon is Irwin, "Cherokee Healing," 237–57. For cultural persistence into the twentieth century, see the works of Jack Kilpatrick and Anna Kilpatrick cited in the bibliography.

29. *Payne-Butrick*, 2:200, 217–18; Mooney, *History, Myths*, 231.

30. Mooney, "Cherokee River Cult," 1–10.

31. Mooney, *History, Myths*, 297.

32. Ibid., 297–300.

33. *Payne-Butrick*, 2:218.

34. Ibid., 1 226, 237, 241, 273; 2:103–104, 153, 218 (quote), 221; Mooney, *History, Myths*, 330–31.

35. Mooney, *Sacred Formulas*, 320.

36. Mooney, *History, Myths*, 251.

37. Ibid., 251; Mooney, *Sacred Formulas*, 361 (quotes).

38. *Payne-Butrick*, 1:226.

39. Ibid., 1:123.

40. Mooney, *History, Myths*, 253.

41. Ibid., 254.

42. *Payne-Butrick*, 1:260.

43. Mooney, *History, Myths*, 253, 295.

44. Ibid., 297.

45. Ibid., 299, 301; *Payne-Butrick*, 1:241.

46. Mooney, *History, Myths*, 298.

47. Olbrechts, ed., *Swimmer Manuscript*, 26; *Payne-Butrick*, 1:239–40.

48. *Payne-Butrick*, 1:240–41.

49. Kelton, "Avoiding the Smallpox Spirits," 49–50; Fogelson, "An Analysis of Cherokee Sorcery and Witchcraft," 113–29.

50. Olbrechts, *Swimmer Manuscript*, 40.

51. Ibid., 28.

52. *Payne-Butrick*, 1:238–39.

53. Ibid., 1:238–39.

54. Ibid., 1:238–41, quote on 241.

55. Olbrechts, *Swimmer Manuscript*, 41.

56. Ibid., 43.

57. Irwin, "Cherokee Healing," 249.

58. Mooney, *History, Myths*, 295.

59. Olbrechts, *Swimmer Manuscript*, 54.

60. *Payne-Butrick*, 1:283; Mooney, *History, Myths*, 240.

61. Irwin, "Cherokee Healing," 248–49.

62. Mooney, *History, Myths*, 240–41; *Payne-Butrick*, 1:214; 2:216, 224.

63. *Payne-Butrick*, 2:216.

64. Ibid., 2:223–24.

65. Olbrechts, *Swimmer Manuscript*, 60.

66. Ibid., 65–66.

67. Adair, *History of the American Indians*, 164; *Payne-Butrick*, 1:256–59; Mooney, *Sacred Formulas*, 330–31.

68. Olbrechts, *Swimmer Manuscript*, 96.

69. Ibid., 98.

70. *Payne-Butrick*, 2:221.

71. Bossu, *Travels in the Interior of North America*, 149.

72. Irwin, "Cherokee Healing," 238.

73. Butrick suggested another ritual called the *E-he-wo-ta-te-gi* or Bounding Bush Ceremony that was practiced in autumn and fixed at the appearance of first moon of the season. His informants told him that this event at some point became less fixed to the seasonal calendar. Description of the ceremony includes a less elaborate set of rituals than other ceremonies. See *Payne-Butrick*, 2:72–73. The Cherokee Nation of Oklahoma notes that "today, many Cherokee traditionalists still observe these festivals. Many ceremonial grounds observe some, and a few observe all of the occasions." See http://www.cherokee.org/AboutTheNation/Culture/General/CherokeeFestivals.aspx (accessed September 23, 2013).

74. *Payne-Butrick*, 1:281–82.

75. Ibid., 1:283.

76. Ibid., 2:150.

77. Ibid., 1:283; Mooney later recorded a similar Cherokee belief: "Of the trees only the cedar, the pine, the spruce, the holly, and the laurel were awake at the end, and to them it was given to always be green and to be greatest for medicine." See Mooney, *History, Myths*, 240.

78. Mooney, "Cherokee River Cult," 1–10.

79. Ibid., 9.

80. *Payne-Butrick*, 1:287–88.

81. Ibid., 2:159.

82. Irwin, "Cherokee Healing," 240.

83. *Payne-Butrick*, 2:143.

84. Hudson, "Why the Southeastern Indians Slaughtered Deer," 155–76.

85. Longe, "Small Postscript," 14.

86. Ibid., 18.

87. Ibid., 40.

88. Ibid., 18.

89. Perdue, *Cherokee Women*, 57–58.

90. Adair, *History of the American Indians*, 252.

91. Ibid., 116.

92. Ibid., 148.

93. Ibid., 151.

94. Moore to [Trustees], September 14, 1739, *CRG*, 5:229.

95. Oglethorpe to Verelst, October 19, 1739, C.O., 5/640/ 399–402 also in *CRG*, 22 (part 2):244–49, quote on 247–48.

96. For a broader treatment of this subject, see Ishii, *Bad Fruits of the Civilized Tree*.

97. *Payne-Butrick*, 1:236.

98. Ibid., 2:229.

99. Ibid., 2:227.

100. Ibid., 2:80.

101. Ibid., 2:229.

102. Adair, *History of the American Indians*, 252–53.

103. *South Carolina Gazette*, June 1, 1738; Marble, *Surgeons, Smallpox, and the Poor*, 7.

104. Adair, *History of the American Indians*, 253–54, 423 (quote).

105. Adair, *History of the American Indians*, 343.

106. *Payne-Butrick*, 1:14.

107. S.C. Council Journal, February [4], 1760, reel 8, RSUS, SC; Perdue, *Cherokee Women*, 29.

108. On physic dance, see *Payne-Butrick*, 2:144, 168.

109. Mooney, *History, Myths*, 421–22.

110. *Payne-Butrick*, 2:225. This reference clearly indicates that practitioners did not think of smallpox as a "whiteman's" disease, which they had no power to combat. Butrick also refers to prayers to prevent measles: "The conj[uror] prays to great beings above called Ni ta we he u, to come and take them away, and send them off to the poplars, (or in the canoes, the phrase being the same)." See *Payne-Butrick*,

2:225–26. The editors of the Butrick papers record that "today *a-ni-da-we-hi-yu* means the 'powerful ones,'" perhaps a reference to guardian spirits of avian creatures. *Payne-Butrick*, 2:227fn.

111. Springplace Diary, June 20, 1824, MAS; Krech, *Spirits of the Air*, 34. The author expresses special thanks to Professor Krech for pointing out the connection between avian creatures and fighting smallpox.

112. Mooney, *History, Myths*, 284; Mooney, *Sacred Formulas*, 334.

113. *Payne-Butrick*, 2:81.

114. Ibid., 2:82.

115. Ibid., 2:229.

116. Grant to Glen, March 5, 1752, *DRIA*, 1:224.

117. Demere to Lyttelton, November 23, 1759, WHL Papers.

118. Richardson Diary, January 14, 1759, NYPL; Timberlake, *Memoirs*, 100–102.

119. Sludders to Devall, May 2, 1749, in Minutes of Council, May 23, 1749, C.O., 5/459/26.

120. Glen to Board of Trade, December 23, 1749, C.O., 5/372/171.

121. Cadogan to Glen, n.d. in Journal of Council, January 18, 1750, C.O., 5/462.

122. Grant and Paxson to Glen, March 23, 1755, *DRIA*, 2:46–47; *South Carolina Gazette*, July 24–31, 1754.

123. Bomer [Beamer] to Glen, April 28, 1755, in *DRIA*, 2:49.

124. Adair, *History of the American Indians*, 166.

125. Ibid., 253.

126. *Payne-Butrick*, 2:53.

127. Adair, *History of the American Indians*, 253.

128. *Payne-Butrick*, 2:221.

129. Norton, *Journal*, 77–78.

130. Haywood, *Natural and Aboriginal*, 266; Hicks to Ross, March 1, 1826, in Moulton, *Papers of Chief John Ross*, 1:115–16.

131. MacGowen, "Indian Secret Societies," 139–41.

132. Mooney, *History, Myths*, 392–93.

133. Fogelson, "Who Were the Ani-Kutani?"

CHAPTER 3

1. Amherst to Montgomery, February 24, 1760, *APSS*, 79–80.

2. Amherst to Lyttelton, February 26, 1760, WHL Papers.

3. Amherst to Bouquet, July 7, 1763, in Stevens et al., eds., *Bouquet Papers*, 6:299–300 (emphasis in the original).

4. Bouquet to Amherst, July 13, 1763, in ibid., ser. 21634, 215.

5. Postscript signed J.A., [Amherst to Bouquet, July 16, 1763], in ibid., 6:315.

6. Trent, "Journal at Fort Pitt, 1763," 400.

7. Quoted in Jones, *Rationalizing Epidemics*, 97.

8. Ibid., 97.

9. Parkman, *Conspiracy of Pontiac*, 44–47, quotes on 44 and 46–47. Even after having access to the Trent journal, which Parkman did not, mid-twentieth century historian Bernhard Knollenberg characterized the Fort Pitt incident as an aberration and irrelevant since he doubted the efficacy of efforts to transmit the virus to indigenous peoples. See Knollenberg, "General Amherst and Germ Warfare"; Knollenberg, "Communications."

10. Mayor, "The Nessus Shirt in the New World," 54–77, quote on 54.

11. Fenn, "Biological Warfare in Eighteenth-Century America," 1552–80, quote 1553.

12. Ward, "The Microbes of War"; Charters, "Military Medicine and the Ethics of War."

13. Vaudreuil to Machault, July 25, 1755, *NYCD* 10:325; "Abstracts of Dispatches received from Canada from Vaudreuil's letters, February 2, 3, 4, 6, 7, & 8 [1756]," *NYCD*, 10:408.

14. Conference between Vaudreuil and the Senecas, October 1, 1755, *NYCD*, 10:345; Williams to Johnson, March 1756, *SWJP* 9:412.

15. Vaudreuil to Minister, August 8, 1756, in Stevens and Kent, eds., *Wilderness Chronicles*, 93–98; Johnson to Loudoun, August 15, 1756, *SWJP*, 9:504; and MacLeod, "Microbes and Muskets," 47.

16. Ward, *Breaking the Backcountry*, 83.

17. Ibid., 150.

18. Shippen to Burd, n.d., Shippen Family Correspondence; Croghan to Johnson, May 7, 1757, *SWJP*, 9:719–20; Johnson to Wraxall, July 17, 1757, *SWJP*, 9:799–800; Johnson's Answer to the Aughquahes, Nanticokes, & other Indians' Speech to him & the Mohocks, August 24, 1757, *SWJP*, 9:813.

19. Bougainville, *Adventure in the Wilderness*, 193 and 197.

20. Ibid., 93–98; Johnson to Loudoun, August 15, 1756, *SWJP*, 9:504.

21. Bougainville, *Adventure in the Wilderness*, 193 and 197 (quotes).

22. Johnson, "Examination of Cornelius Van Slyke," July 21, 1767, quoted in Fenn, "Biological Warfare in Eighteenth-Century America," 1566. For a larger discussion of the politics of disease in New France during the Seven Years' War, see MacLeod, "Microbes and Muskets."

23. Blackbird, *History of the Ottawa and Chippewa*, 9–10.

24. Ibid., 10.

25. Intelligence from Judge's Friend to Demere, December 10, 1756, *DRIA*, 2:265.

26. Demere to Lyttelton, April 2, 1757, *DRIA*, 2:358.

27. Talk of Oxinaa to Demere, April 8, 1757, *DRIA*, 2:411–12.

28. Lyttelton to Board of Trade, December 25, 1756, *BPROSC*, 27:209.

29. Demere to Lyttelton, January 15, 1757, *DRIA*, 2:315.

30. Boggs to Lyttelton, February 21, 1757, *DRIA*, 2: 343; Dobbs to Lyttelton, April 10, 1757, WHL Papers.

31. Kelton, "The British and Indian War."

32. St. Clair to Forbes, May 19, 1758, Forbes Papers, reel 2, item 234; Byrd to Lachlin Mackintosh, May 12, 1758, Tinling, ed., *Correspondence of the Byrds*, 2:665;

Minutes of Virginia Council in ibid; Attakullakulla to Byrd, May 27, 1758, in ibid., 656–57; Callaway to Washington, May 15, 1758, Abbot et al., eds., *Papers of George Washington*, 5:183; Depositions Concerning Indian Disturbances in Virginia, June 1, 1758, *DRIA*, 2:463–70; St. Clair to Blair, May 31, 1758, Abbot et al., *Papers of George Washington*, 5:197; Byrd to Forbes, May 21, 1758, Forbes Papers, reel 2, item 239.

33. St. Clair to Forbes, May 24, 1758, ibid., reel 2.

34. St. Clair to Forbes, May 25, 1758, ibid., reel 2.

35. St. Clair to Bouquet, June 9, 1758, Stevens et al., *Bouquet Papers*, 2:61–62.

36. Bouquet to Forbes, June 14, 1758 and June 16, 1758, in ibid., 2:87–89 and 95.

37. Bouquet to Forbes, June 16, 1758, in ibid., 2:95–96.

38. Bouquet to Washington, July 14, 1758, Abbot et al., *Papers of George Washington*, 5:287; Bouquet to Forbes, July 15, 1758, Stevens et al., *Bouquet Papers*, 2:215–17.

39. Memorandum of James Beamer, April 20, 1758, *DRIA*, 2:451–52. Whether the trader actually said this is not certain. The headmen of the Middle Town of Cowee claimed that lies were being told about him. See Talk of Headmen of Cowee to Lyttelton, May 12, 1758, WHL Papers.

40. Cherokee Warriors to Lyttelton, April 13, 1758, *DRIA*, 2:452–53.

41. Statement to President Blair, June 22, 1758, Draper Mss., Virginia Papers, 4ZZ, 52.

42. Turner to [Forbes?], June 23, 1758, Forbes Papers, reel 2, item 325.

43. Turner to [Byrd], June 23, 1758, ibid., reel 2, item 326.

44. Turner to Lyttelton, July 2, 1758, *DRIA*, 2:471.

45. Turner to Lyttelton, July 2, 1758, *DRIA*, 2:471.

46. Lyttelton to Atkin, June 10, 1758, Letter book, WHL Papers; Atkin to Howarth, June 21, 1758, WHL Papers.

47. Lloyd to Atkin, June 25, 1758, WHL Papers; *South Carolina Gazette*, July 7, 1758.

48. Mackintosh to Lyttelton, August 7, 1758, Letter book, WHL Papers.

49. Richardson Diary, January 14, 1759, NYPL.

50. Demere to Lyttelton, February 26, 1759, WHL Papers.

51. On the origins of the Anglo-Cherokee War, see Oliphant, *Peace and War*, 69–112.

52. Amherst to Lyttelton, December 21, 1759, WHL Papers.

53. Dobbs to Lyttelton, October 11, 1759, ibid.

54. Lyttelton to Dobbs, October 19, 1759, Letter book, ibid.

55. Richardson to M.J.F., May 6, 1760, Davies, *Letters*, 21. Richardson reported on his activities of a year earlier so the epidemic occurred in May 1759.

56. Virginia Council Minutes, June 4, 1759, Tinling, *Correspondence of the Byrds*, 2:674.

57. Talk sent from King Hagler and other Catawbas, October 1759, WHL Papers.

58. Wyly to Lyttelton, November 5, 1759, ibid.

59. *South Carolina Gazette*, December 15, 1759.

60. Coytmore to Lyttelton, November 11, 1759, WHL Papers.

61. Adair, *History of the American Indians*, 267–68.

62. Coytmore to Lyttelton, December 3, 1759, and December 6, 1759, WHL Papers.

63. *South Carolina Gazette*, December 22, 1759. Oliphant believes that of this number, only 1,300 were effective due to desertion and disease. See Oliphant, *Peace and War*, 109.

64. *South Carolina Gazette*, December 8, 1759.

65. Ibid., December 22, 1759, and January 12, 1760.

66. First Conference with Attakullakulla or the Little Carpenter and the Cherokee Warrior with him at Fort Prince George on the 18th December 1759, WHL Papers.

67. Second Conference with Attakullakulla & the Cherokee Warriors with him at Ft. Prince George on the 19th December 1759, ibid.

68. *South Carolina Gazette*, January 12, 1760.

69. Corkran, *Cherokee Frontier*, 188.

70. Adair, *History of the American Indians*, 265.

71. Lyttelton to Council, December 29, 1759, in S.C. Council Journal, January 8, 1760, reel 8, RSUS, SC.

72. John Stuart to Allan [Stuart], May 15, 1760, James Grant Papers, reel 31.

73. Lyttelton to Board of Trade, December 29, 1759, *BPROSC*, 28:284; *South Carolina Gazette*, January 12, 1760; Milligan, "A Short Description," 525–26; William Fyffe to John Fyffe, February 1, 1761, Thomas Gilcrease Museum, typed ms. The epidemic in South Carolina is discussed in Kresbach, "The Great Charlestown Smallpox Epidemic of 1760." Oliphant calls this "Lyttelton's folly." See Oliphant, *Peace and War*, 108–10.

74. Milne to Lyttelton, February 24, 1760, *DRIA*, 2: 501.

75. Fort Prince George Journal, January 17, 1760, W.O., 34/35, LOC transcripts.

76. Fort Prince George Journal, February 1, 1760, W.O., 34/35, ibid.; Oliphant, *Peace and War*, 110.

77. Fort Prince George Journal, February 3–5, 1760, W.O., 34/35, LOC transcripts.

78. Coytmore to Lyttelton, February 7, 1760, WHL Papers.

79. Fort Prince George Journal, February 8, 1760, ibid.

80. Fort Prince George Journal, February 8–24, 1760, ibid.

81. Corkran, *Cherokee Frontier*, 196–98.

82. Ibid., 192–93.

83. Francis to Lyttelton, March 6, 1760, *DRIA*, 2:504.

84. Fort Prince George Journal, February 14, 1760, WHL Papers.

85. Corkran, *Cherokee Frontier*, 195.

86. Milne to Lyttelton, February 24, 1760, *DRIA*, 2:497, 499–500.

87. Fort Prince George Journal, February 16, 1760, WHL Papers; Adair, *History of the American Indians*, 267.

88. Adair, *History of the American Indians*, 267. Oliphant agrees with Adair's assessment and calls Milne's account "too theatrical to require comment." See Oliphant, *Peace and War*, 111.

89. Lyttelton to Amherst, [n.d. c. February 20, 1760], Letter book, WHL Papers.

90. *Maryland Gazette*, May 8, 1760.

91. Montgomery to Amherst, April 12, 1760, *APSS*, 90–93.

92. Lyttelton to Ellis, February 4, 1760, WHL Papers.

93. Milligan, "A Short Description," 528; Bull to Amherst, May [16?], 1760, W.O., 34/35, LOC transcripts.

94. House of Assembly, February 10, 1760, WHL Papers.

95. S.C. Council Journal, February 29, 1760, reel 8, RSUS, SC.

96. Corkran, *Cherokee Frontier*, 201.

97. S.C. Council Journal, May 6, 1760, reel 8, RSUS, SC.

98. Ellis to Board of Trade, February 15, 1760, C.O., 5/647/5.

99. South Carolina Council, April 22, 1760, reel 9, RSUS, SC.

100. Ellis to Board of Trade, May 15, 1760, C.O., 5/648/3.

101. Coytmore to Lyttelton, January 7, 1760, WHL Papers.

102. *South Carolina Gazette*, January 19, 1760.

103. Fort Prince George Journal, February 3, 1760, W.O., 34/35, LOC transcripts.

104. *South Carolina Gazette*, April 19, 1760 (emphasis in the original).

105. Ibid., April 7, 1760.

106. Montgomery to Amherst, April 12, 1760, *APSS*, 90–93.

107. Lyttelton to Amherst, February 2, 1760 and February 9, 1760, Letter book, WHL Papers.

108. Lyttelton to Amherst, February 18, 1760, Letter book, ibid.

109. Amherst to Montgomery, February 24, 1760, *APSS*, 79–80.

110. Amherst to Montgomery, March 6, 1760, ibid., 83; Transports for South Carolina March 14, 1760, ibid., 88.

111. *South Carolina Gazette*, June 14, 1760. In this edition, the *Gazette* printed various extracts of letters sent back to Charles Town but does not provide the names of those who provided these dispatches.

112. Montgomery to Amherst, June 4, 1760, *APSS*, 123.

113. *South Carolina Gazette*, June 10, 1760. The newspaper reprinted a letter Grant sent to Bull, June 4, 1760, which can be found in S.C. Council Journal, June 10, 1760, reel 8, RSUS, SC.

114. *South Carolina Gazette*, June 14, 1760.

115. Amherst to Montgomery, June 29, 1760, *APSS*, 124.

116. Montgomery to Amherst, June 23, 1760, ibid., 125.

117. Bull to Board of Trade, June 30, 1760, *BPROSC*, 28:365.

118. For details on the Battle of Etchoe, see Oliphant, *Peace and War*, 130–32.

119. Montgomery to Amherst, July 2, 1760, *APSS*, 128–29.

120. S.C. Council Journal, August 11, 1760, reel 8, RSUS, SC.

121. *Pennsylvania Gazette*, September 4, 1760.

122. *South Carolina Gazette*, June 21, 1760, September 27, 1760.

123. Ibid., October 18, 1760.

124. Ibid., October 25, 1760.

125. S.C. Council Journal, October 22, 1760, reel 8, RSUS, SC.

126. Bull to Board of Trade, June 30, 1760, *BPROSC*, 28:365; *South Carolina Gazette*, July 5, 1760.

127. Bull to Board of Trade, June 30, 1760, *BPROSC*, 28:365–66; *South Carolina Gazette*, August 2, 1760, and October 18, 1760.

128. *South Carolina Gazette*, October 25, 1760.

129. Ibid., February 7, 1761.

130. Ibid., January 24, 1761; January 31, 1761.

131. *Maryland Gazette*, November 27, 1760.

132. *South Carolina Gazette*, January 31, 1761.

133. Grant to Amherst, June 2, 1761, *APSS*, 267; Bull to Board of Trade, June 19, 1761, *BPROSC*, 29:119.

134. *Pennsylvania Gazette*, September 4, 1760 (emphasis in original). This report was reprinted in *Maryland Gazette*, September 11, 1760.

135. Corkran, *Cherokee Frontier*, 219–22.

136. Amherst to Bull, October 14, 1760, W.O., 34/36, PRO reel 241; Bull to Amherst, October 19, 1760, W.O., 34/35, LOC transcripts.

137. Amherst to Bull, extract November 27, 1760, James Grant Papers, reel 31.

138. Amherst to Bull, November 27, 1760, ibid., reel 31.

139. Amherst to Grant, December 15, 1760, *APSS*, 150–51.

140. Grant to Amherst, December 20, 1760, ibid., 160.

141. [Amherst] to Grant, December 21, 1760, ibid., 163.

142. *South Carolina Gazette*, May 23, 1761; Oliphant, *Peace and War*, 147.

143. *South Carolina Gazette* April 25, 1761.

144. Ibid., May 9, 1761.

145. Grant to Bull, June 2, 1761, James Grant Papers, reel 32; Grant to Amherst, June 2, 1761, *APSS*, 267.

146. Grant's Talk to Little Carpenter, May 23, 1761, *APSS*, 262–63.

147. French, "Journal of an Expedition," 287.

148. Ibid., 284.

149. *Maryland Gazette*, August 13, 1761.

150. French, "Journal of an Expedition," 284; Grant, "Journal," 30.

151. *South Carolina Gazette*, July 18, 1761, and September 5, 1761. Grant's campaign is detailed in Oliphant, *Peace and War*, 159–163.

152. Grant, "Journal," 26.

153. Amherst to Grant, August 1, 1761, *APSS*, 288.

154. A Letter Signed Philolethes [March 2, 1763], Hamer, ed., *Papers of Lauren*, 3:286.

155. French, "Journal of an Expedition," 288.

156. *Maryland Gazette*, September 10, 1761; "A Letter Signed Philolethes [March 2, 1763]," Hamer, *Papers of Lauren*, 3:342.

157. Attakullakulla to Byrd, July 7, 1761, Tinling, *Correspondence of the Three Byrds*, 2:745.

158. Attakullakulla's Talk to Col. Grant, August 29, 1761, *APSS*, 293 (quote) and 294; Grant to [Bull], September 2, 1761, James Grant Papers, reel 32. See also Little Carpenter to Bull in S.C. Council Journal, September 15, 1761, reel 8, RSUS, SC.

159. A Letter Signed Philolethes [March 2, 1763], Hamer, *Papers of Lauren*, 3:286.

160. Grant to Amherst, September 3, 1761, *APSS*, 301.

161. Grant to Amherst, September 3, 1761, ibid., 301 (quote); Grant to Bull, September 2, 1761, James Grant Papers, reel 32.

162. Amherst to Grant, October 2, 1761, *APSS*, 309.

163. "Report by Arthur Dobbs concerning general conditions in North Carolina, 1761," *CSRNC*, 6:616–17.

164. Adair, *History of the American Indians*, 248.

165. Wood, "Changing Population of the Colonial South," 65.

166. Axtell, for example, cautions against the use of genocide when explaining what happened to Natives, claiming that "the vast majority of Indians succumbed . . . to new and lethal epidemic diseases imported *inadvertently* by the settlers." He adds that "only one or two verifiable instances" of deliberate germ warfare occurred. Axtell, *Beyond 1492*, 262. A more strident critic of the idea that what happened to American Indians constitutes genocide is Steven T. Katz, who uncritically cites epidemics to make his case that the vast majority of Native deaths did not involve the agency of colonizers and were thus unintended. See Katz, "Uniqueness," 20–22. It is unfortunate that the "virgin soil" thesis has tied scholarly hands when it comes to assessing the degree to which colonizers perpetrated crimes against humanity against indigenous peoples of the Americas.

CHAPTER 4

1. Donelson, "Journal of a Voyage" (accessed October 29, 2013).

2. Brown to Cornwallis, December 17, 1780, *CP*, 3:296.

3. Clements, "An Analysis of 'the Original' Donelson Journal." In 1844, Lyman Draper made a handwritten copy of the "original" journal and it remains in the Draper Manuscript Collection of the Wisconsin Historical Society.

4. Fleming, "Journal," 642.

5. Donelson, "Journal of a Voyage."

6. Carr, *Early Times in Middle Tennessee*, 9.

7. Carr to Draper, October 10, 1854, Draper Mss., 6XX, 63.

8. Haywood, *Natural and Aboriginal History of Tennessee*, 85–96; Ramsey, *The Annals of Tennessee*, 197–202.

9. Carr, *Early Times in Middle Tennessee*, 9.

10. Putnam, *History of Middle Tennessee*, 69–77, quote on 77.

11. Putnam, *History of Middle Tennessee*, 77; Adair, *History of the American Indians*, 253.

12. Putnam, *History of Middle Tennessee*, 77.

13. Ibid., 309.

14. Roosevelt, *Winning of the West*, 2:336–37.

15. Ibid., 2:337.

16. Mooney, *History, Myths*, 56.

17. Brown, *Old Frontiers*, 182n9.

18. Stearn and Stearn, *The Effect of Smallpox*, 8 (quote) and 46.

19. Two examples include Peter Wood, who cites Brown's 1938 book, and Russell Thornton, who cites the Stearns' work, to support the claim that smallpox struck Cherokees in 1780. See Wood, "The Impact of Smallpox," 35; Thornton, *The Cherokees*, 34.

20. Fenn, *Pox Americana*, 116.

21. Ibid., 133.

22. Ibid., 275.

23. Stuart to Amherst, October 4, 1763, W.O., 34/47; Cochrane to Bull, November 10, 1764, Gage Papers, vol. 25; Cameron to Price, March 16, 1765, enclosed in Cochrane to Gage, April 26, 1765, Gage Papers, vol. 35; Cochrane to Gage, June 3, 1765, Gage Papers, vol. 37; Cameron to Stuart, April 9, 1766, C.O., 5/66/396.

24. Perdue, "Cherokee Relations with the Iroquois," 143; Dowd, *War under Heaven*, 77, 226–27, 263–64.

25. Congress at Fort Prince George, May 8, 1766, enclosed in Stuart to Gage, August 2, 1766, Gage Papers, vol. 55.

26. Phillips to Gage, June 14, 1766, Gage Papers, vol. 52; Talk of Cherokees to Stuart, August 22, 1766, C.O., 5/67/244.

27. Phillips to Gage, September 24, 1766, Gage Papers, vol. 57.

28. Talk of Kittagusta to Stuart, September 22, 1766, C.O., 5/67/240.

29. Phillips to Gage, January 22, 1767, Gage Papers, vol. 61.

30. Talk of Kittagusta to Stuart, September 22, 1766, C.O., 5/67/240.

31. Stuart to Faquier, November 24, 1766, C.O., 5/67/212.

32. John David Hammerer, Report on the Cherokees, September 26, 1766, MAB, Box 191, fo. 3, item 1.

33. Phillips to Gage, October 16, 1766, Gage Papers, vol. 58.

34. Stuart to Gage, December 19, 1766, ibid., vol. 60.

35. Stuart to Gage, July 21, 1767, ibid., vol. 67.

36. Keough to Gage, October 24, 1767, ibid., vol. 71.

37. Stuart to Gage, May 17, 1768, vol. 77; Cameron to Stuart, April 21, 1768, vol. 77; Cameron to Stuart, May 20, 1768, vol. 78; Stuart to Gage, July 2, 1768, vol. 78; Talk of the Headmen and Warriors of the Cherokee Nation to Stuart, July 29, 1769, vol. 87; all in ibid.

38. Proceedings of Cherokees at Congarees, April 1770, ibid., vol. 137.

39. Stuart to Gage, January 27, 1770, vol. 89; Stuart to Gage, December 12, 1770, vol. 98; Stuart to Gage, February 8, 1771, vol. 99; all in ibid.

40. Stuart to Gage, April 29, 1771, ibid., vol. 102.

41. Cameron to Stuart, [February 8], 1771, ibid., vol. 100.

42. Stuart to Gage, December 25, 1773, ibid., vol. 119.

43. Extract of Cameron to Stuart, November 2, 1772, ibid., vol. 119.

44. Abstract of Cameron to Stuart, December 30, 1772, ibid., vol. 116; Stuart to Gage, December 25, 1773, ibid., vol. 119.

45. Cameron to Stuart, June 18, 1774, ibid., vol. 120.

46. Talks from Lower Cherokees, February 21, 1774, C.O., 5/75/83.

47. Cameron to Stuart, March 1, 1774, C.O., 5/75/70.

48. Stuart to Gage, May 12, 1774, Gage Papers, vol. 119.

49. Talk of Judd's Friend [Ostenaca] to Governor of South Carolina, November 3, 1762, reel 8, RSUS, SC.

50. Hatley, "The Three Lives of Keowee," 223–48.

51. Wood, "Changing Population of the Colonial South," 38 and 65.

52. A useful overview of the larger experience of indigenous peoples during the Revolutionary War can be found in Schmidt, *Native Americans in the American Revolution*.

53. Journal of Superintendent [John Stuart]'s proceedings at Hard Labor, September 28–October 17, 1768, Gage Papers, vol. 137.

54. Talk of the Headmen & Warriors of the Cherokee Nation to Stuart, July 29, 1769, ibid., vol. 87.

55. Proceedings of Cherokees at Congarees, April 1770, ibid., vol. 137.

56. Faragher, *Daniel Boone*, 92–96.

57. Campbell to Cameron, June 20, 1774, Gage Papers, vol. 123.

58. Cumfer, *Separate Peoples, One Land*, 28–29.

59. Piecuch, *Three Peoples, One King*, 65–66.

60. Lower Cherokees Speech to Party Setting off for East Florida, November 8, 1775, C.O., 5/77/85.

61. O'Donnell, *Southern Indians in the American Revolution*, 33.

62. Blackmon, *Dark and Bloody Ground*, 45.

63. Henry Stuart to John Stuart, August 25, 1776, *CSRNC* 10:763–85.

64. O'Donnell, *Southern Indians in the American Revolution*, 42–43.

65. Creswell to Drayton, July 27, 1776, in Gibbes, ed., *Documentary History*, 2:30–31; Blackmon, *Dark and Bloody Ground*, 55–56.

66. Preston to Fleming, July 25, 1776, Draper Mss., 1U26.

67. Cameron to Stuart, May 7, 1776, C.O., 5/77/139; Norton, *Journal*, 41 and 57.

68. Hatley, *The Dividing Paths*, 192.

69. Jefferson to Pendleton, August 13, 1776, the Avalon Project, Documents in Law, History and Diplomacy, http://avalon.law.yale.edu/18th_century/let8.asp (accessed October 25, 2013).

70. Purdie to Fleming, August 18, 1776, Draper Mss., 1U32.

71. Drayton to Salvador, July 24, 1776, in Gibbes, *Documentary History*, 2:28–30, quote on 29.

72. Rutherford to North Carolina Council of Safety, July 5, 1776, *CSRNC*, 10:651–52, quote on 652.

73. Rockwell, "Parallel and Combined Expeditions," 214.

74. Ibid., 214.

75. William Williams Affidavit (R11628), RWP.

76. Moore to Rutherford, November 17, 1776, *CSRNC*, 10:895–98, quote 897.

77. Rockwell, "Parallel and Combined Expeditions," 219.

78. Ibid., 219–20; Hamilton, ed., "Revolutionary Diary of William Lenoir," 256.

79. William Christian to Patrick Henry, October 15, 1776, in "Virginia Legislative Papers," 61.

80. Christian to Henry, October 15, 1776, in ibid., 60.

81. Christian to Henry, October 15, 1776, in ibid., 62.

82. Christian to Henry, October 15, 1776, in ibid., 62.

83. Williams to President of the Provincial Congress of North Carolina, *CSRNC*, 10:892.

84. Williams, ed., "Colonel Joseph Williams' Battalion," 110–11.

85. Cherokee deaths to violence are unknowable, although one historian without citing a source puts the number of dead at two thousand. (See Lumpkin, *From Savannah to Yorktown*, 25.) This number seems too high given that most Cherokees abandoned their towns, but not necessarily too high if death from starvation and exposure are considered. In any event, those numbers are unknowable as well.

86. O'Donnell, *Southern Indians in the American Revolution*, 57–58.

87. Charles Stuart to John Stuart, April 8, 1777, C.O., 5/78/128.

88. Stuart to Germain, March 5, 1778, C.O., 5/79/134.

89. Talk from the Raven to Governor Caswell, April 14, 1778, *CSRNC*, 13:90–91.

90. Cashin, *The King's Ranger*, 83–84.

91. Stuart to Germaine, January 11, 1779, C.O., 5/80/76; Stuart to Principal Chiefs, Head mean, and Warriors of the Upper and Lower Creeks, February 1, 1779, C.O., 5/80/244; John Stuart to Taitt, February 1, 1779, C.O., 5/80/248.

92. Talk of the Cowee Warrior to Stuart, [c. March 1779], C.O., 5/80/175.

93. Jefferson to Washington, June 19, 1779, *PTJ*, 3:6; Extract of a Letter from Grierson to Taitt, May 24, 1779, C.O., 5/80/250.

94. Cameron to Germain, December 18, 1779, HQP, 20:2489.

95. Calloway places the evacuation of Chickamauga Creek and construction of five new towns farther down the Tennessee in 1779 following Shelby's campaign. The weight of the evidence, which will be discussed later, indicates that abandonment of Chickamauga Creek occurred in 1782. See Calloway, *American Revolution in Indian Country*, 203.

96. Cameron to Hamilton, July 15, 1779, Haldimand Papers, 1777–83.

97. Chiefs of Chuccamogga to Evan Shelby, May 21, 1779, Thomas Jefferson Papers, LOC, http://memory.loc.gov/cgi-bin/query/P?mtj:10:./temp/~ammem _ZBtK (accessed May 9, 2013).

98. Norton, *Journal*, 42–43.

99. Fenn, *Pox Americana*, 111.

100. Papers of the Continental Congress, NARA, RG 360, M247, reel 85, item 71, p. 265, in Fold3, http://www.fold3.com/s.php#query=Cherokee&offset=11&prev iew=1&t=63 (accessed April 27, 2013).

101. Campbell to Clinton, February 10, 1779, HQP, 15:1737.

102. Board of Commissioners to Head Men and Warriors in the Great Tallassie, June 6, 1779, C.O., 5/81/271.

103. Cameron to Prevost, October 15, 1779, C.O., 5/182/207.

104. *Pennsylvania Gazette*, October 17, 1779.

105. Cameron's 1779 letters, in which one would think he would mention an epidemic among the Cherokees but did not, include: Cameron to Hamilton, July 15, 1779, Haldimand Papers, 1777–83; Cameron to Prevost, October 15, 1779, C.O., 5/182/207; Cameron to Germaine, December 18, 1779, HQP, 20:2489.

106. Williamson to Lincoln, September 22, 1779, BLP, reel 4. Williamson reports eight towns destroyed; the British reported he destroyed six. (See Cameron to Prevost, October 15, 1779, C.O., 5/182/207.)

107. John Morgan, S7243, RWP.

108. Cameron to Prevost, October 15, 1779, C.O., 5/182/ 207.

109. Cameron to Germaine, December 18, 1779, HQP, 20:2489.

110. Coffee to Eaton, December 30, 1829, NARA, RG 75, M234, reel 73.

111. Presentments of a Respectable Grand Jury of Georgia March 1780, in *The Papers of Lachlan McIntosh*, 12:87.

112. Brown to Germain, March 10, 1780, Savannah, C.O., 5/81/155.

113. Clinton to Prevost, March 8, 1780, HQP, 22:2621.

114. Brown to Germain, March 18, 1780, C.O., 5/81/161.

115. Prevost to Clinton, March 19, 1780, HQP, 22:2647.

116. Brown to Cornwallis, December 17, 1780, *CP*, 3:295–97. If a smallpox epidemic had raged to the extent that historians have claimed, one would also think American documents would have referenced the event. But no mention can be found in such documents. See Arthur Campbell to William Campbell, August 13, 1780, in Kellogg, ed., *Frontier Retreat*, 24:244–45; [Unknown to unknown], September 22, 1780, Draper Mss., 16DD12; Deposition of William Springstone, December 11, 1780, *CVSP*, 1:446–47.

117. McArthur to Cornwallis, *CP*, 3:330; Campbell to Jefferson, February 28, 1781, *PTJ*, 5:20.

118. Martin to Jefferson, December 12, 1780, *PTJ*, 4:200–201.

119. Campbell to Jefferson, January 15, 1781, *PTJ*, 4:359–63, quotes 361.

120. Campbell, Sevier, and Martin to Chiefs and Warriors of the Cherokees, January 4, 1781, *CVSP*, 1:414–15.

121. Campbell to Jefferson, February 28, 1781, *PTJ*, 5:20; Blackmon, *Dark and Bloody Ground*, 186–91.

122. Campbell to Jefferson, March 28, 1781, *PTJ*, 5:267–68.

123. Martin to Jefferson, March 31, 1781, *PTJ*, 5:304–305.

124. Talk Delivered by Clanosee or the Horse Leach & Aucoo, Messengers sent by Oconostotee & some other Chiefs of the Cherokee Nation, April 28, 1781, Draper Mss., 1XX43.

125. Talk of Cherokee Nation delivered by the Raven of Chottee, September 1, 1781, C.O., 5/82/287.

126. Brown to Germain, April 6, 1782, C.O., 5/82/277.

127. Pickens to Greene, July 19, 1781, 9:48–50; Pickens to Greene, July 25, 1781, 9:77–78; Bryan to Greene, August 27, 1781, 9:260–61, quote on 260; all in *Greene Papers*.

128. Extract of a Letter from Colo[nel] E. Clarke, November 15, 1781, in Keith Read Collection, University of Georgia, online http://neptune3.galib.uga.edu/ssp/cgi-bin/tei-natamer-idx.pl?sessionid=7f000001&type=doc&tei2id=krc067 (accessed May 9, 2013).

129. Pickens Campaign of 1781, Draper Mss., 3VV142–46.

130. Brown to Earl of Shelburne, September 25, 1782, *DAR*, 20:122–23, quote on 122.

131. Browne to [Leslie], December 5, 1781, HQP, 33:3930; Vann to Martin, December 21, 1781, enclosed in Shelby to Campbell, December 31, 1781, Virginia, Governor's Office Letters Received, Library of Virginia, online, http://image.lva.virginia.gov/GLR/02845/ (accessed January 27, 2014).

132. Ferguson, "General Andrew Pickens," 258–59.

133. Stevens, *History of Georgia*, 2:285.

134. Pickens to Clark, January 25, 1782, Thomas Addis Emmet Collection, NYPL, http://archives.nypl.org/collection/1#id3309 (accessed May 23, 2013).

135. Ibid.

136. Pickens to Clarke, April 3, 1782, in Stevens, *History of Georgia*, 2:283–85.

137. No firsthand accounts of McDowell's March 1782 campaign are known to exist. Participants later recalled the campaign but offered few details. See RWP, Hodge (W4234), Withrow (S6403), and Davidson (S1758). See also Blackmon, *Dark and Bloody Ground*, 221.

138. Shelby to Campbell, April 29, 1782, Virginia, Governor's Office Letters Received, Library of Virginia, online, http://image.lva.virginia.gov/GLR/03364/ (accessed June 25, 2013).

139. Campbell to Edmondson, September 13, 1782, Draper Mss. 9DD38; Cashin, *The King's Ranger*, 155.

140. Pickens to Greene, September 7, 1782, *Greene Papers*, 11:633–34, quote on 634.

141. Pickens to Martin, October 26, 1782, Miscellaneous American, Literary, and Historical Manuscripts, Pierpont Morgan Library, New York.

142. Moses Perkins (S3677), RWP.

143. Brown to Ramsey, December 25. 1786, in White, ed., *Historical Collections of Georgia*, 2:614–19, quote on 614.

144. Pickens to Lee, August 28, 1811, Draper Mss., 1VV107.

145. A third prong of the fall 1782 campaign may have happened but the sources are not entirely clear. Joseph McDowell was ordered by Alexander Martin to attack the Valley Towns but no report of a campaign exists and postwar recollections of Revolutionary War veterans are too vague or contradictory to piece together what happened. See Martin to McDowell, July 23, 1782, *CSRNC* 16:697–98. Abraham Forney (W3976), RWP.

146. Sevier, "Memoir." This memoir contains essentially the same information that James related in his affidavit to receive a veteran's pension. See James Sevier (S45889), RWP.

147. Quotes taken from pension affidavits in RWP in order: William Coleman (S3196); Jesse Byrd (R1574); Tidence Lane (W377); Bowling Baker (S12950); David Hall (S1823). See also William Smith (S1723) and John Crabb (R2417)

148. Christian to Harrison, December 16, 1782, *CVSP*, 3:398.

149. Brown to Carleton, January 12, 1783, HQP, 60:6742.

150. For an analysis of this post–Revolutionary War violence, see Cumfer, *Separate Peoples, One Land*.

151. Wood, "Changing Population in the Colonial South," 38.

152. Jones, "Virgin Soils Revisited"; Cameron et al, ed. *Beyond Germs*.

153. Jones, "Death, Uncertainty, and Rhetoric."

CHAPTER 5

Epigraph Source: Bloomfield, *Good Tidings*, 31.

1. Jenner to Dunning, May 17, 1802, in Baron, *Life of Jenner*, 330–31, quote on 331.

2. "An Account of the First Festival of the Royal Jennerian Society for the Extermination of the Small-Pox, on Thursday, May 17, 1803," *Gentleman's Magazine*, May 1803, 463.

3. Bloomfield, *Good Tidings*, 30–31.

4. The story of Jenner's life and work is well-known. For an overview of his life and work, see Fisher, *Edward Jenner, 1749–1823*.

5. Waterhouse to Jenner, April 8, 1802, in Halsey, *How the President*, 55 (emphasis in original). Waterhouse included essentially the same story in a letter to his colleague J. C. Lettsom who in turn had the letter published in a widely circulated periodical. Jenner may have also read this letter, but it did not refer to the Cherokees being those vaccinated or among the embassy. See "To the Editor of the European Magazine," *European Magazine*, 41 (April 1802): 246. The vaccination of Little Turtle is also reported in *Independent Chronicle*, May 20, 1802, vol. 34, no. 2206. This story was later reprinted with some revisions in *Christian Observer* 1, no. 8 (August 1802): 536, wherein the chief is called "Little Pigeon" and the editors added the comment, "Such was the confidence of the Indians in their more civilized neighbors, that all the warriors caused themselves to be inoculated."

6. The most thorough overview of this time period is McLoughlin, *Cherokee Renascence*. See also Perdue, *Cherokee Women*; Miles, *House on Diamond Hill*.

7. On the origins of the U.S. government's "civilization" policy, see Sheehan, *Seeds of Extinction*; and Wallace, *Jefferson and the Indians*.

8. Norton, *Journal*, 157.

9. Meigs to Eustis, December 1, 1809, NARA, RG 75, M208, reel 4. For an assessment of this census, see Thornton, *The Cherokees*, 47–48.

10. Wood, "Changing Population in the Colonial South," 38.

11. *BJ*, 74; Hoyt et al. to Worcester, July 25, 1818, ABCFM, reel 73.

12. Perdue, *Cherokee Women*, 108–84.

13. Ross et al. to Monroe, January 19, 1824, Moulton, *Papers of Chief John Ross*, 1:61.

14. For a broader theoretically informed discussion of this political development, see Champagne, *Social Order and Political Change*. On the role of slavery in this development, see Perdue, *Slavery and the Evolution of Cherokee Society*.

15. McLoughlin, *Cherokees and Missionaries*, 157, 167, and 175.

16. On early nineteenth-century U.S. medicine, see Valenčius, *The Health of the Country*, 54–69 and 74–78.

17. On healthcare provided to the Vanns, see entries of Springplace Diary, dated July 6, October 16, 1802; February 24, March 5, August 14–15, 1803; August 19, 1804; and entries in *MSMC*, 2:8, 119, 126, 142, 205, 220.

18. Examples not discussed below can be found in October 1, 1803 entry of Diary of Wohlfahrt and Byham, MAB, Box 193, fo. 3; *MSMC*, 2:208, 253, 362, 426.

19. *MSMC*, 1:335.

20. Ibid., 1:351.

21. Ibid., 1:410.

22. Ibid., 1:568–69.

23. Ibid., 2:147.

24. Ibid., 1:205.

25. Ibid., 2:173.

26. Ibid., 1:119.

27. Ibid., 1:354, 362, 373, 423.

28. Ibid., 1:368.

29. Ibid., 1:483.

30. Ibid., 1:332–35.

31. Ibid., 2:31 and 36.

32. October 25, 1822, and January 11, 1823, Springplace Diary.

33. *MSMC*, 2:237, 238, 246, 247.

34. Ibid., 2:116.

35. Ibid., 1:483. The diary entry reads "our Dick's mother." The student was Dick Dyeentohee, whose mother was Goadi. See ibid., 2:460 and 462.

36. Ibid., 1:332, 333–34, 335.

37. Ibid., 1:351.

38. Ibid., 2:220–21.

39. Ibid., 2:385.

40. January 9 and April 21, 1824, Springplace Diary.

41. *BJ*, 217, 506fn21.

42. *MSMC*, 1:562. Gu'ulisi is referred to in the Moravian records by his English name, "Big Halfbreed."

43. Ibid., 2:110 (emphasis in original).

44. Ibid., 2:463.

45. McLoughlin, *Cherokee Renascence*, 358, 378–79.

46. *BJ*, 217, 225, 227, 235, 282.

47. Butler to Evarts, June 21, 1822, ABCFM, reel 738.

48. *BJ*, 280; Butler to Evarts, August 13, 1823, ABCFM, reel 738.

49. *BJ*, 281.

50. *BJ*, 272–73.

51. *BJ*, 284.

52. Butler to Evarts, January 12, 1823, ABCFM, reel 738.

53. *BJ*, 345.

54. *BJ*, 384.

55. Elsworth to Evarts, August 25, 1823, ABCFM, reel 738.

56. Elsworth to Evarts, n.d. [probably 1824], ibid., reel 739.

57. "Inventory of Items at Taloney, November 22, 1819," ibid., reel 738.

58. June 10, 11, and 14, 1822, Moody Hall Journal, ibid., reel 738.

59. September 2, 3, and 4, 1822, Moody Hall Journal, ibid., reel 738.

60. See his journal entries for December 4 and 10, 1822; June 14 and 28, 1823; July 15, 1823; September 27–28, 1823, October 11, 1823, in Moody Hall Journal, ibid., reel 738.

61. July 16, 1823, Moody Hall Journal, ibid., reel 738.

62. August 23, 1823, Moody Hall Journal, ibid., reel 738.

63. August 2, 1823, Moody Hall Journal, ibid., reel 738.

64. Hall to Evarts, May 25, 1820, reel 738; November 24, 1822, Moody Hall Journal, ibid., reel 738.

65. May 17, 1822, Moody Hall Journal, ibid., reel 738.

66. November 5, 1822, Moody Hall Journal, ibid., reel 738.

67. William Chamberlain, Private Journal, ibid., reel 738.

68. Butrick to Evarts, October 25, 1823, ibid., reel 738.

69. Proctor to Evarts, July 28, 1827, ibid., reel 739; [?] to Evarts, August 20, 1829, ibid., reel 739.

70. Potter to Evarts, June 29, 1824, ibid., reel 739.

71. For this incident, see entries dated April 26, 27, 28 and May 4, 10, 30, 1824 in Moody Hall Journal, ibid., reel 738.

72. Chiefs of Eu-hal-la to Hicks and Pathkiller, May 26, 1824, MAS, [signed by Chuleoa, Aolenaugait, Shoe Boots, Canul lahut, Cannetohut, Ca Che ta use, Eyausoo, Hanta tago, written by Wallis Adair]. The Moravians commented in general on the animosity toward missionaries at Hightower. See Schmidt to Schulz, June 7, 1824, MAS; Anna and John Gambold to Schultz, July 22, 1824, MAS.

73. Chamberlain to Evarts, July 30, 1824, ABCFM, reel 739.

74. Minutes of a Conference between Secretary of War and a Deputation of Cherokees, June 30, 1801 and July 3, 1801, NARA, RG 75, M15, reel 1; *National Intelligencer and Washington Advertiser*, July 15, 1801; Jefferson to Martha Jefferson, July 16, 1801, *TJP*, 34:580.

75. On the introduction of smallpox vaccine to the United States, see Halsey, *How the President*; Blake, *Benjamin Waterhouse*.

76. Jefferson to Waterhouse, July 25, 1801, in Founders Archives, online, http://founders.archives.gov/?q=Author%3A%22Jefferson%2C%20Thomas%22%20Recipient%3A%22Waterhouse%2C%20Benjamin%22&s=1111311111&r=3&sr=Waterhouse (accessed December 18, 2013); Jefferson to Waterhouse, August 14, 1801, http://founders.archives.gov/?q=Author%3A%22Jefferson%2C%20Thomas%22%20Recipient%3A%22Waterhouse%2C%20Benjamin%22&s=1111311111&r=5&sr=Waterhouse (accessed December 18, 2013).

77. For more on this subject, see Pearson, "Medical Diplomacy and the American Indian."

78. Records of the Cherokees meeting with Jefferson in Washington, D.C., make no mention of receiving cowpox, but Hicks would later report that he was indeed vaccinated. On the Cherokees' trip to Washington, D.C., see documents in NARA, RG 75, M15, reel 2, frames 59–71.

79. Hicks to Meigs, March 3, 1806, NARA, RG 75, M208, reel 3.

80. Blackburn to Chairman of the Standing Committee of Missions [Ashbel Green], January 27, 1806, in *The General Assembly's Missionary Magazine; or Evangelical Intelligencer* 2 (January 1806): 137.

81. Miles, *The House on Diamond Hill*, 4–5.

82. Pathkiller and Lowery to Meigs, February 17, 1806, in Tennessee Documentary History, online http://diglib.lib.utk.edu/cgi/t/text/pageviewer-idx?c=tdh;cc=tdh;sid=9ec75e321064128910898db308481d85;q1=Meigs;idno=pa0018;seq=00000003 (accessed January 9, 2014).

83. Glass, Justice, Boggs, & Hicks to Meigs, March 5, 1806, in Tennessee Documentary History, online, http://diglib.lib.utk.edu/cgi/t/text/pageviewer-idx?c=tdh;cc=tdh;sid=9ec75e321064128910898db308481d85;q1=Meigs;idno=pa0203;seq=1;view=image;size=s (accessed January 9, 2014).

84. Cherokee Agency Journal, April 9, 1806, NARA, RG 75, M208, reel 11; Cherokee Day Book, 1801–1810, entry for October 27, 1808, NARA, RG 75, M208, reel 12.

85. Ross to Meigs, March 24, 1806, in Tennessee Documentary History, online, http://diglib.lib.utk.edu/cgi/t/text/pageviewer-idx?c=tdh;cc=tdh;sid=9ec75e321064128910898db308481d85;q1=Meigs;idno=pa0019;seq=00000002 (accessed January 9, 2014).

86. Blackburn to Green, June 9, 1806, in *The General Assembly's Missionary Magazine; or Evangelical Intelligencer*, 2 (September 1806): 494–495, quote 495.

87. Committee of Missions, Philadelphia, March 13, 1806, Daniel Parker Papers, Box 13, fo. 9.

88. Blackburn to Green, June 9, 1806, in *General Assembly's Missionary Magazine; or Evangelical Intelligencer* 2 (September 1806): 494–95.

89. *MSMC*, 1:149, 168–69.

90. Ibid., 1:149; Byhan to Reichel, December 5, 1806, MAS.

91. *BJ*, 197. In 1821, Reverend Ard Hoyt of the ABCFM paid Dr. Strong one hundred dollars for unspecified reasons, although it could have been for the previous year's vaccination. Hoyt to Evarts, March 31, 1821, ABCFM, reel 738.

92. *Western Carolinian*, May 11, 1824.

93. *Augusta Chronicle*, July 3, 1824; June 11, 1824, Springplace Diary.

94. June 11, 1824, Springplace Diary.

95. June 20, 1824, ibid.

96. Moulton, *John Ross, Cherokee Chief*, 6–7 and 15–28.

97. Schmidt to Schultz, July 13, 1824, MAS.

98. *Augusta Chronicle*, July 3, 1824; *Carolina Observer*, July 22, 1824.

99. Schmidt to Schultz, July 13, 1824, MAS.

100. July 10, 1824, Springplace Diary.

101. July 11, 1824, ibid.

102. Schmidt to Schultz, July 13, 1824, MAS.

103. July 10, 1824, Springplace Diary.

104. McLoughlin, *Cherokees and Missionaries*, 392.

105. June 21, 1824, Springplace Diary.

106. Hall to Evarts, June 29, 1824, ABCFM, reel 738.

107. Hall to Evarts, June 29, 1824, ibid., reel 738.

108. Moody Hall Journal, July 9, 1824, ibid., reel 738.

109. Hicks to McMinn, September 26, 1824, M234, reel 71.

110. Dawson's letter was published in *Latter Day Luminary* 5 (1824): 281; Jones's letter was published in *Baptist Missionary Magazine* 5 (1825): 153. Lack of evidence prior to 1826 prevents an analysis of the Valley Towns region to determine whether the same pattern of medical pluralism was developing there. McLoughlin's work, however, suggests that such pluralism developed as the work of Evan Jones intensified during the 1820s and 1830s. See McLoughlin, *Champions of the Cherokees*, 64–96.

111. Hall to Evarts, July 28, 1824, ABCFM, reel 738.

112. William Chamberlain Journal, December 1824, ibid., reel 739.

113. *Christian Advocate and Journal and Zion's Herald*, 4 no. 11 (November 13, 1829).

114. Butrick to Evarts, October 18, 1824, ABCFM, reel 739.

115. Proctor to Evarts, July 28, 1827, ibid., reel 739.

116. December 30, 1830, Butrick Journal, ibid., reel 754.

117. [N.d.], Butrick Journal, ibid., reel 754.

Conclusion

1. The results of the census are appended to Cherokee National Council, *Laws of the Cherokee Nation* (accessed December 9, 2013).

2. One of the agents involved in conducting the 1824 census estimated the numbers that moved in from North Carolina and those who at the time of the census lived in the West. See *Cherokee Phoenix and Indians' Advocate*, February 24, 1830, online through Western Carolina University, Hunter Library, http://www.wcu.edu/library/DigitalCollections/CherokeePhoenix/V012/n045/pg2c014a-pg2c011b.htm (accessed January 30, 2014).

3. Adair, *History of the American Indians*, 249. Adair received his information from "the most intelligent old traders," who lived among the Cherokees for several decades. These traders probably included Robert Bunning, Cornelius Doherty, James Beamer, and Ludovick Grant. See Memorial of Robert Bunning and Others, November 22, 1751, *DRIA*, 1:148.

4. An Address from the friendly Chiefs of the Cherokees to the Commissioners of the United States, April 29, 1782, *CVSP*, 3:171–72.

5. Talk from the Little Turkey and the Headmen and Warriors of the Overhill Cherokees to Brown, November 17, 1783, C.O., 5/82/446. Savanukeh carried the talk to Florida where he recited it to Brown.

6. The demographic impact of Cherokee removal is more fully discussed in Thornton, *The Cherokees*, 73–76.

7. A succinct and well-done treatment of Cherokee removal is Perdue and Green, *The Cherokee Nation and the Trail of Tears*.

8. William Chamberlain Journal, October–November, 1824, ABCFM, vol. 4, reel 739.

9. McLoughlin, *Cherokees and Missionaries*, 186.

BIBLIOGRAPHY

ARCHIVES

Amherst, Jeffery. Papers. War Office Records 34. National Archives of the United Kingdom (formerly known as the British Public Record Office). Transcripts and microfilm at Library of Congress, Washington, D.C.

Colonial Office Records. National Archives of the United Kingdom (formerly known as the British Public Record Office). Transcripts.

Fyffe, William, to John Fyffe. Typescript ms., February 1, 1761. Thomas Gilcrease Museum of American Art and History, Tulsa, Okla.

Gage, General Thomas. Papers. William L. Clements Library, University of Michigan, Ann Arbor.

Letters. Moravian Archives, Salem, N.C.

Lyttelton, William Henry. Papers. William L. Clements Library, University of Michigan, Ann Arbor.

Miscellaneous American, Literary, and Historical Manuscripts. Pierpont Morgan Library, New York.

Parker, Daniel. Papers. Historical Society of Pennsylvania, Philadelphia.

Richardson, William. Diary. New York Public Library, New York.

Shippen Family Correspondence. Historical Society of Pennsylvania, Philadelphia.

Springplace Diary and Correspondence. Moravian Archives, Salem, N.C.

Traunter, Richard. "Travels between Virginia and South Carolina, 1698–1699." Typescript. Virginia Historical Society, Richmond, Va. (provided by Wendy St. Jean).

MICROFILM COLLECTIONS

American Board of Commissioners for Foreign Missions Records. Houghton Library, Harvard University, Cambridge, Mass.

British Headquarters. (Sir Guy Carleton) Papers. Colonial Williamsburg Foundation, Williamsburg, Va.

Colonial Office Records. National Archives of the United Kingdom (formerly known as the British Public Record Office), Library of Congress, and Hunter Library, Western Carolina University, Cullowhee, N.C.

Draper, Lyman Copeland. Manuscripts. Wisconsin Historical Society, Madison.

Grant, James, of Ballindalloch. Papers. National Archives of Scotland, Edinburgh.

Haldimand, Sir Frederick. Unpublished Papers and Correspondence, 1758–84. British Museum, London.

Headquarters Papers of General John Forbes Relating to the Expedition against Fort Duquesne. University of Virginia Library, Charlottesville.

Journal of the Commons House of Assembly of South Carolina. Transcripts. South Carolina Department of History and Archives, Columbia.

Lincoln, Benjamin. Papers. Massachusetts Historical Society, Boston.

Moravian Mission Records among the North American Indians. Moravian Archives, Bethlehem, Pa.

Office of Indians Affairs. Letters Received, 1824–81. National Archives and Records Administration, Washington, D.C. RG 75 (M234).

Records in the British Public Records Office Relating to South Carolina. Transcribed by W. Noel Sainsbury. 36 vols. South Carolina Department of History and Archives, Columbia.

Records of the Cherokee Agency in Tennessee. National Archives and Records Administration, Washington, D.C. RG 75 (M208).

Records of the Society for the Propagation of the Gospel. Society for the Propagation of the Gospel in Foreign Parts, London.

Records of the States of the United States of America. Library of Congress, Washington, D.C.

Secretary of War. Letters Sent Relating to Indian Affairs, 1800–1824. National Archives and Records Administration, Washington, D.C. RG 75 (M15).

Newspapers and Periodicals

Augusta (Ga.) Chronicle
Baptist Missionary Magazine (Boston)
Carolina Observer (Fayetteville, N.C.)
Cherokee Phoenix and Indians' Advocate (New Echota, Cherokee Nation)
Christian Advocate and Journal and Zion's Herald (New York)
Christian Observer (London)
European Magazine (London)
General Assembly's Missionary Magazine; or Evangelical Intelligencer (Philadelphia)
Gentleman's Magazine (London)
Latter Day Luminary (Philadelphia)
Maryland Gazette (Annapolis)
National Intelligencer and Washington Advertiser (Washington, D.C.)

Pennsylvania Gazette (Philadelphia)
South Carolina Gazette (Charleston)
Western Carolinian (Asheville, N.C.)

DIGITAL COLLECTIONS

Avalon Project. Documents in Law, History and Diplomacy. Yale University Law
    School. http://avalon.law.yale.edu/.
Donelson, John. "Journal of a Voyage," transcript. Tennessee State Library and
    Archives. http://www.tn.gov/tsla/founding_docs/33635_Transcript.pdf.
Emmet, Thomas Addis, Collection. New York Public Library, New York. http://
    archives.nypl.org/collection/1#id3309.
Founders Archives. National Archives and Records Administration. http://found-
    ers.archives.gov.
Jefferson, Thomas. Papers. Library of Congress, American Memory. http://memory
    .loc.gov.
Papers of the Continental Congress. NARA, RG 360, Fold3. http://www.fold3.com/.
Read, Keith, Collection. Digital Library of Georgia. University of Georgia Library,
    Athens. http://dlg.galileo.usg.edu/.
Revolutionary War Pension and Bounty—Land Warrant Application Files. National
    Archives and Records Administration, RG 15, Fold3. http://www.fold3.com/.
Tennessee Documentary History. http://diglib.lib.utk.edu/dlc/tdh/index.html.

PUBLISHED PRIMARY SOURCES

Abbot, W. W., Dorothy Twohig, and Chase Philander, eds. *The Papers of George
    Washington. Colonial Series*. 10 vols. Charlottesville: University Press of Vir-
    ginia, 1983–95.
Adair, James. *The History of the American Indians*. Edited by Kathryn Holland Braund.
    Tuscaloosa: University of Alabama Press, 2005.
Alvord, Clarence Walworth, and Lee Bidgood, eds. *The First Explorations of the
    Trans-Allegheny Region by the Virginians, 1650–1674*. Cleveland: Arthur H. Clark
    Company, 1912.
American State Papers: Indian Affairs. Vol. 1. Washington, D.C.: Gales and Seaton, 1832.
Anderson, William L., Anne F. Rogers, and Jane L. Brown, eds. *The Payne-Butrick
    Papers*. 2 vols. Lincoln: University of Nebraska Press, 2010.
Baron, John, ed. *The Life of Edward Jenner: With Illustrations of his Doctrines, and
    Selections from his Correspondence*. London: H. Colburn, 1827–38.
Bloomfield, Robert. *Good Tidings; or, News from the Farm*. London: Parnassian
    Press, 1804.
Boyd, Julian P., Lyman H. Butterfield, and Mina R. Bryan, eds. *Papers of Thomas
    Jefferson*. Vols. 3–5. Princeton, N.J.: Princeton University Press, 1951–52.

Bossu, [Jean-Bernard]. *Travels in the Interior of North America, 1751–1762*. Edited and translated by Seymour Feiler. Norman: University of Oklahoma Press, 1962.

Bougainville, Louis Antoine de. *Adventure in the Wilderness: The American Journals of Louis Antoine de Bougainville, 1756–1760*. Edited and translated by Edward P. Hamilton. Norman: University of Oklahoma Press, 1964.

Boyd, Mark F., trans. "The Expedition of Marcus Delgado from Apalachee to the Upper Creek Country in 1866." *Florida Historical Quarterly* 16 (January 1937): 3–48.

Brock, R. A., ed. *The Official Letters of Alexander Spotswood*. 2 vols. Richmond: Virginia Historical Society, 1882.

Byrd, William, II. *The Writings of Colonel William Byrd of Westover in Virginia*. Edited by John Spencer Bassett. New York: Doubleday, Page, and Company, 1901.

Candler, Allen, Lucian Knight, Kenneth Coleman, and Milton Ready, eds. *Colonial Records of the State of Georgia*. 39 vols. Atlanta: Franklin Printing and Publishing; Athens: University of Georgia Press, 1904–.

Cherokee National Council. *Laws of the Cherokee Nation [1808–1824]*. Online through Library of Congress, American Indian Constitutions and Legal Materials, http://www.loc.gov/law/help/american-indian-consts/PDF/28014184.pdf.

"Cherokee Traditions." *Cherokee Phoenix* 11, no. 3 (April 1, 1829).

Chicken, George. "A Journal from Carolina in 1715 [1716]." In *Yearbook of the City of Charleston*, 324–54. Charleston, S.C.: Walker, Erono, and Cogswell, 1894.

Clayton, Langdon, and Vernon Knight, eds. *The De Soto Chronicles: The Expedition of Hernando de Soto to the United States, 1539–1543*. 2 vols. Tuscaloosa: University of Alabama, 1993.

Cuming, Alexander. "Journal of Sir Alexander Cuming (1730)." In *Early Travels in the Tennessee Country, 1540–1800*, edited by Samuel Cole Williams, 115–46. Johnson County, Tenn.: Watauga Press, 1928.

Davies, Kenneth G., ed. *Documents of the American Revolution, 1770–1783*. 21 vols. Dublin: Irish University Press, 1972–81.

Davies, Samuel. *Letters from the Rev. Samuel Davis &c: Shewing the State of Religion (Particularly among the Negroes) in Virginia*. London: 1757.

Fleming, William. "Journal of Travels in Kentucky, 1779–1780." In *Travels in the American Colonies*, edited by Newton D. Mereness, 617–55. New York: MacMillan Company, 1916.

French, Christopher. "Journal of an Expedition to South Carolina." *Journal of Cherokee Studies* 2 (Summer 1977): 275–301.

Gibbes, Robert W., ed. *Documentary History of the American Revolution*. 3 vols. New York: D. Appleton and Co., 1857; Spartanburg, S.C. Reprint Company, 1972.

Grant, James. "Journal of Lieutenant-Colonel James Grant, Commanding an Expedition against the Cherokee Indians, June–July, 1761." *Florida Historical Quarterly* 12 (July 1933): 25–36.

Grant, Ludovick. "Historical Relation of Facts Delivered by Ludovick Grant, Indian Trader, to His Excellency the Governor of South Carolina." *South Carolina Historical and Genealogical Magazine* 10 (January 1909): 54–68.

Hamer, Philip M., ed. *The Papers of Henry Laurens*. 16 vols. Columbia: University of South Carolina Press, 1968–2003.

Hamilton, J. G. de Roulhac, ed. "Revolutionary Diary of William Lenoir." *Journal of Southern History* 6 (May 1940): 247–59.

Hann, John, trans. "Translation of Governor Robolledo's 1657 Visitation of Three Florida Provinces and Related Documents." *Florida Archaeology* 2 (1986): 81–145.

Hawes, Lilla M., ed. *The Papers of Lachlan McIntosh, 1774–1779*. Collections of the Georgia Historical Society. Vol. 12. Savannah: Georgia Historical Society, 1957.

———. *The Proceedings and Minutes of the Governor and Council of Georgia, October 4, 1774, through November 7, 1775 and September 6, 1779 through September 20, 1780*. Collections of the Georgia Historical Society. Vol. 10. Savannah: Georgia Historical Society, 1957.

Heckewelder, John. *A Narrative of the Mission of the United Brethren among the Delaware and Mohegan Indians*. Philadelphia: McCarty and Davis, 1820.

Henderson, Archibald, ed. "The Treaty of Long Island of Holston, July 1777." *North Carolina Historical Review* 8 (January 1931): 58–117.

Hudson, Charles, ed., and Paul E. Hoffman, trans. *The Juan Pardo Expeditions: Exploration of the Carolinas and Tennessee, 1566–1568*. Washington, D.C.: Smithsonian Institution Press, 1990.

Kellogg, Louise Phelps, ed. *Frontier Advance on the Upper Ohio, 1778–1779*. Collections of the Wisconsin Historical Society. Vol. 23. Madison: Wisconsin Historical Society, 1916.

———. *Frontier Retreat on the Upper Ohio, 1779–1781*. Collections of the Wisconsin Historical Society. Vol. 24. Madison: Wisconsin Historical Society, 1917.

Klingberg, Frank, ed. *The Carolina Chronicle of Dr. Francis Le Jau*. University of California Publications in History, vol. 53. Berkeley: University of California Press, 1956.

———, ed. *Carolina Chronicle: The Papers of Gideon Johnston*. University of California Publications in History. Vol. 35. Berkeley: University of California Press, 1946.

Lane, Mills, ed. *General Oglethorpe's Georgia: Colonial Letters, 1733–1743*. 2 vols. Savannah: Beehive Press, 1975.

Le Moyne d'Iberville, Pierre. *Iberville's Gulf Journals*. Edited and translated by Richebourg Gaillard McWilliams. Tuscaloosa: University of Alabama Press, 1981.

Longe, Alexander. "A Small Postscript on the Ways and Manners of the Indians Called Cherokees [c.1711]." *Southern Indian Studies* 21 (October 1969): 6–49.

Mays, Edith, ed. *Amherst Papers, 1756–1763, The Southern Sector: Dispatches from South Carolina, Virginia and His Majesty's Superintendent of Indian Affairs*. Westminster, Md.: Heritage Books, 2006.

McClinton, Rowena, ed. *The Moravian Springplace Mission to the Cherokees*. 2 vols. Lincoln: University of Nebraska Press, 2007.

McDowell, William L., ed. *Journals of the Commissioners of the Indian Trade, September 20, 1710–August 29, 1718*. Columbia: South Carolina Archives Department, 1955.

———, ed. *Documents Relating to Indian Affairs, 1750–1754*. Columbia: South Carolina Archives Department, 1958.

————, ed. *Documents Relating to Indian Affairs, 1754–1765*. Columbia: University of South Carolina Press, 1970.

McCrady, Edward. *History of South Carolina*. 4 vols. New York: MacMillan, 1897–1902.

Milligan, George. "A Short Description of the Province of South Carolina with an Account of the Air, Weather, and Diseases, at Charles-Town Written in the Year 1763." In *Historical Collections of South Carolina: Embracing Many Rare and Valuable Pamphlets, and Other Documents, Relating to the History of that State from its First Discovery to its Independence, in the Year 1776*, edited by Bartholomew Rivers Carroll, 463–535. New York: Harper and Bros., 1836.

Moore, Alexander, ed. *Nairne's Muskhogean Journals: The 1708 Expedition to the Mississippi River*. Jackson: University Press of Mississippi, 1988.

Moulton, Gary, ed. *The Papers of Chief John Ross*. 2 vols. Norman: University of Oklahoma Press, 1985.

Norton, John. *The Journal of Major John Norton, 1816*. Edited by Carl F. Klinck and James J. Talman. 1970. Reprint, Toronto: Champlain Society, 2011.

O'Callaghan, Edmund, John Brodhead, and Berthold Fernow, eds. *Documents Relative to the Colonial History of the State of New York*. 15 vols. Albany: Weed, Parsons, and Company, 1853–87.

Palmer, William, Sherwin McRae, Raleigh Edward Colston, and Henry W. Flournoy, eds. *Calendar of Virginia State Papers and Other Manuscripts*. 11 vols. Richmond: Virginia State Library, 1875–93.

Pénicaut, André. *Fleur de Lys and Calumet: Being the Pénicaut Narrative of French Adventure in Louisiana*. Translated and edited by Richebourg Gaillard McWilliams. Tuscaloosa: University of Alabama Press, 1987.

Phillips, Joyce B., and Paul Gary Phillips, eds. *The Brainerd Journal: A Mission to the Cherokees, 1817–1823*. Lincoln: University of Nebraska Press, 1998.

Robinson, Thomas B. "An Indian King's Will." *Virginia Magazine of History and Biography* 36 (April 1928): 192–93.

Rockwell, E[lijah] F., ed. "Parallel and Combined Expeditions against the Cherokee Indians in South and in North Carolina in 1776." *Historical Magazine* 2nd Series, 2 (October 1867): 212–20.

Rowland, Dunbar, A. G. Sanders, and Patricia Galloway, eds. *Mississippi Provincial Archives, French Dominion*. 5 vols. Jackson: Mississippi Department of Archives and History, 1927–32 and 1984.

Saberton, Ian, ed. *The Cornwallis Papers*. 6 vols. East Sussex, U.K.: Naval and Military Press, 2010.

Salley, Alexander S., ed. *Commissions and Instructions from the Lords Proprietors of Carolina to Public Officials of South Carolina, 1685–1715*. Columbia: South Carolina Department of History and Archives, 1916.

————, ed. *The Journal of the Commons House of Assembly of South Carolina*. 21 vols. Columbia: South Carolina Department of Archives and History, 1907–49.

————, ed. *Narratives of Early Carolina, 1650–1708*. New York: Charles Scribner's Sons, 1911.

Saunders, William L., and Walter Clark, eds. *The Colonial and State Records of North Carolina*. 26 vols. Raleigh: P. M. Hale, 1886–1907.

Schwartz, Stuart B., ed. *Victors and Vanquished: Spanish and Nahua Views of the Conquest*. New York: Macmillan, 2000.

Sevier, James. "A Memoir of John Sevier." *American Historical Magazine* 6 (January 1901): 40–45.

Shea, John D., ed. *Early Voyages up and down the Mississippi by Cavelier, St. Cosme, Le Seur, Gravier, and Guignas*. Albany: Joel Munsell, 1861.

Showman, Richard, ed. *The Papers of General Nathanael Greene*. 13 vols. Chapel Hill: University of North Carolina Press, 1976–2005.

Stevens, Sylvester, and Donald H. Kent, eds. *Wilderness Chronicles of Northwestern Pennsylvania*. Harrisburg: Pennsylvania Historical Commission, 1941.

Stevens, Sylvester, Donald H. Kent, Autumn L. Leonard, L. M. Waddell, and J. L. Tottenham, eds. *The Papers of Colonel Henry Bouquet*. 18 vols. Harrisburg: Pennsylvania Historical and Museum Commission, 1940–43.

Sullivan, James, Alexander C. Flick, Almon W. Lauber, and Milton W. Hamilton, ed. *The Papers of Sir William Johnson*. 14 vols. Albany: University of the State of New York, 1921–65.

Tennessee Historical Commission, ed. *Three Pioneer Tennessee Documents: Donelson's Journal, Cumberland Compact, Minutes of Cumberland Court*. Knoxville: University of Tennessee Press, 1964.

Timberlake, Henry. *Lieutenant Henry Timberlake's Memoirs, 1756–1765*. Edited by Samuel Cole Williams. New York: Arno Press, 1971.

Tinling, Marion, ed. *The Correspondence of the Three William Byrds of Westover, Virginia, 1684–1776*. 2 vols. Charlottesville: University Press of Virginia, 1977.

Trent, William. "William Trent's Journal at Fort Pitt, 1763." Edited by Albert T. Volwiler. *Mississippi Valley Historical Review* 11 (December 1924): 390–413.

Vassar, Rena, ed. "Some Short Remarkes on the Indian Trade in the Charikees and in Management thereof since the Year 1717." *Ethnohistory* 8 (Autumn 1961): 401–23.

"Virginia Legislative Papers." *Virginia Magazine of History and Biography* 17 (January 1909): 52–64.

White, George. *Historical Collections of Georgia*. Vol. 2. New York: Pudney and Russell, 1854.

Williams, Joseph. "Colonel Joseph Williams' Battalion in Christian's Campaign." Edited by Samuel C. Williams. *Tennessee Historical Magazine* New series, 9 (April 1925): 102–16.

Williams, Samuel Cole, ed. *Early Travels in the Tennessee Country, 1540–1800*. Johnson County, Tenn.: Watauga Press, 1928.

Winthrop, John. *1631–1637*. Vol. 3 of *Winthrop Papers*. Boston: Massachusetts Historical Society, 1943.

Worth, John, ed. and trans. *The Struggle for the Georgia Coast: An 18th-Century Spanish Retrospective on Guale and Mocama*. Anthropological Papers of the American Museum of Natural History, no. 75. Athens: University of Georgia Press, 1995.

SECONDARY SOURCES

Ackerknect, Erwin. *History and Geography of the Most Important Diseases.* New York: Hafner, 1965.

Alchon, Suzanne. *A Pest in the Land: New World Epidemics in a Global Perspective.* Albuquerque: University of New Mexico Press, 2003.

Anderson, David. "Stability and Change in Chiefdom-Level Societies: An Examination of Mississippian Political Evolution on the South Atlantic Slope." In *Lamar Archaeology*, edited by Gary Shapiro, 187–252. Tuscaloosa: University of Alabama Press, 1987.

Aquila, Richard. *The Iroquois Restoration: Diplomacy on the Colonial Frontier, 1701–1754.* Lincoln: University of Nebraska Press, 1997.

Axtell, James. *Beyond 1492: Encounters in Colonial North America.* New York: Oxford University Press, 1992.

———. *The Invasion Within: The Contest of Cultures in Colonial North America.* New York: Oxford University Press, 1985.

———. *Natives and Newcomers: The Cultural Origins of North America.* New York: Oxford Unviersity Press, 2001.

Barquet, Nicolau, and Pere Domingo. "Smallpox: The Triumph over the Most Terrible of the Ministers of Death." *Annals of Internal Medicine* 127 (1997): 635–42.

Beck, Robin A., Jr., "From Joara to Chiaha: Spanish Exploration of the Appalachian Summit." *Southeastern Archaeology* 16 (Winter 1997): 162–69.

Beck, Robin A., Jr., and David G. Moore. "The Burke Phase: A Mississippian Frontier in the North Carolina Foothills." *Southeastern Archaeology* 21 (Winter 2002): 192–205.

Beck, Robin A., Jr., David G. Moore, and Christopher B. Rodning. "Conflict, Violence, and Warfare in *La Florida*." In *Native and Spanish New Worlds: Sixteenth-Century Entradas in the American Southwest and Southeast,* edited by Clay Mathers, Jeffrey Mitchem, and Charles Haecker, 232–49. Amerind Studies in Anthropology. Tucson: University of Arizona Press, 2013.

———. "Identifying Fort San Juan: A Sixteenth-Century Spanish Occupation at the Berry Site, North Carolina." *Southeastern Archaeology* 25 (Summer 2006): 65–77.

———. "Limiting Resistance: Juan Pardo and the Shrinking of Spanish La Florida, 1566–1568." In *Enduring Conquests: Rethinking the Archaeology of Resistance to Spanish Colonialism in the Americas,* edited by Matthew Liebmann and Melissa S. Murphy, 19–39. Santa Fe, N. Mex.: School for Advanced Research Press, 2011.

Blackbird, Andrew J. *History of the Ottawa and Chippewa Indians in Michigan.* Ypsilanti, Mich.: Ypsilantian Job Printing House, 1887.

Blackhawk, Ned. *Violence over the Land: Indians and Empires in the Early American West.* Cambridge, Mass.: Harvard University Press, 2006.

Blackmon, Richard D. *Dark and Bloody Ground: The American Revolution along the Southern Frontier.* Yardley, Pa.: Westholme Publishing, 2012.

Blake, John Ballard. *Benjamin Waterhouse and the Introduction of Vaccination: A Reappraisal.* Philadelphia: University of Pennsylvania Press, 1957.

Blanton, Wyndham B. *Medicine in Virginia in the Seventeenth Century.* Richmond, Va.: William Byrd Press, 1930.

Blitz, John H. *Ancient Chiefdoms of the Tombigbee.* Tuscaloosa: University of Alabama Press, 1993.

Boulware, Tyler. *Deconstructing the Cherokee Nation: Town, Region, and Nation among the Eighteenth-Century Cherokees.* Gainesville: University Press of Florida, 2011.

Bowne, Eric E. *The Westo Indians: Slave Traders of the Early Colonial South.* Tuscaloosa: University of Alabama Press, 2005.

Brown, John P. *Old Frontiers: The Story of the Cherokee Indians from Earliest Times to the Date of Their Removal to the West, 1838.* Kingsport, Tenn.: Southern Publishers, 1938.

Calloway, Colin G. *American Revolution in Indian Country: Crisis and Diversity in Native American Communities.* New York: Cambridge University Press, 1995.

————. *New Worlds for All: Indians, Europeans, and the Remaking of Early America.* Baltimore, Md.: Johns Hopkins University Press, 1997.

Cameron, Catherine, Paul Kelton, and Alan Swedlund, eds. *Beyond Germs: Explorations of Native Depopulation in North America.* Tucson: University of Arizona Press, forthcoming.

Carr, John. *Early Times in Middle Tennessee.* Nashville: E. Stevenson and F. A. Owen, 1857.

Cashin, Edward J. *The King's Ranger: Thomas Brown and the American Revolution on the Southern Frontier.* Athens: University of Georgia Press, 1989.

Champagne, Duane. *Social Order and Political Change: Constitutional Governments among the Cherokee, the Choctaw, the Chickasaw, and the Creek.* Stanford, Calif.: Stanford University Press, 1992.

Chapman, Jefferson. *Tellico Archaeology: 12,000 Years of Native American History.* Knoxville: University of Tennessee Press, 1985.

Charters, Erica. "Military Medicine and the Ethics of War: British Colonial Warfare during the Seven Years War (1756–63)." *Canadian Bulletin for the History of Medicine* 27 (December 2010): 273–98.

Chin, James, ed. *Control of Communicable Diseases Manual.* 17th ed. Washington, D.C.: American Public Health Association, 2000.

Churchill, Ward. *A Little Matter of Genocide: Holocaust and Denial in the Americas 1492 to Present.* San Francisco, Calif.: City Light Books, 1997.

Clements, Paul. "An Analysis of 'the Original' Donelson Journal and Associated Accounts of the Donelson Party Voyage." *Tennessee Historical Quarterly* 64 (Winter 2005): 339–49.

Cook, Noble David. *Born to Die: Disease and New World Conquest, 1492–1650.* Cambridge, N.Y.: Cambridge University Press, 1998.

Cooper, Donald, and Kenneth Kiple. "Yellow Fever." In *Cambridge World History of Human Disease,* edited by Kennth Kiple, 1100–107.

Corkran, David. *The Cherokee Frontier: Conflict and Survival, 1754–62.* Norman: University of Oklahoma Press, 1962.

Crane, Verner. *The Southern Frontier, 1670–1732.* Ann Arbor: University of Michigan Press, 1929.

Cronon, William. *Changes in the Land: Indians, Colonists, and the Ecology of New England*. New York: Hill and Wang, 1983.

Crosby, Alfred. *Ecological Imperialism: The Biological Expansion of Europe, 900–1900*. New York: Cambridge University Press, 1986.

———. "Virgin Soil Epidemics as a Factor in the Aboriginal Depopulation in America." *William and Mary Quarterly* 3rd ser., 33 (April 1976): 289–99.

Cumfer, Cynthia. *Separate Peoples, One Land: The Minds of Cherokees, Blacks, and Whites on the Tennessee Frontier*. Chapel Hill: University of North Carolina, 2007.

Daniels, John D. "The Indian Population of North America in 1492." *William and Mary Quarterly* 3rd ser. 49 (April 1992): 298–320.

DePratter, Chester "The Chiefdom of Cofitachequ." In *The Forgotten Centuries: Indians and Europeans in the American South, 1521–1704*, edited by Charles Hudson and Carmen Chaves Tesser, 197–226. Athens: University of Georgia, 1994.

Diamond, Jared. *Guns, Germs, and Steel: The Fates of Human Societies*. New York: W. W. Norton, 1997.

Dickens, Roy S. *Cherokee Prehistory: The Pisagah Phase in the Appalachian Summit Region*. Knoxville: University of Tennessee Press, 1976.

———. "Mississippian Settlement Patterns in the Appalachian Summit Area: The Pisgah and Qualla Phases." In *Mississippian Settlement Patterns*, edited by Bruce D. Smith, 115–40. New York: Academic Press, 1978.

Dickson, Bruce D. "Yanomamö of the Mississippi Valley? Some Reflections on Larson (1972) and Gibson (1974) and Mississippian Warfare in the Southeastern United States." *American Antiquity* 46 (October 1981): 909–16.

Dobyns, Henry. "Estimating Aboriginal American Population: An Appraisal of Techniques with a New Hemispheric Estimate," *Current Anthropology* 7 (September 1966): 395–416.

———. *Their Number Become Thinned: Native American Population Dynamics in Eastern North America*. Knoxville: University of Tennessee Press, 1983.

Dowd, Gregory Evans. *War under Heaven: Pontiac, the Indian Nations, & the British Empire*. Baltimore, Md.: Johns Hopkins University Press, 2002.

Emerson, Thomas E. *Cahokia and the Archaeology of Power*. Tuscaloosa: Unviersity of Alabama Press, 1997.

Ethridge, Robbie, and Charles Hudson, eds. *Transformation of the Southeastern Indians: 1540–1760*. Jackson: University Press of Mississippi, 2002.

Ethridge, Robbie, and Sheri M. Shuck-Hall, ed. *Mapping the Mississippian Shatter Zone*. Lincoln: University of Nebraska Press, 2009.

Faragher, John Mack. *Daniel Boone: The Life and Legend of an American Pioneer*. New York: Holt, 1992.

Fenn, Elizabeth. "Biological Warfare in Eighteenth-Century North America: Beyond Jeffrey Amherst," *Journal of American History* 86 (March 2000): 1552–80.

———. *Pox Americana: The Great Smallpox Epidemic of 1775–82*. New York: Hill and Wang, 2001.

Ferguson, Clyde A. "General Andrew Pickens." PhD diss., Duke University, 1960.

Fisher, Edward. *Edward Jenner, 1749–1823*. London: André Deutsch, 1991.

Fogelson, Raymond D. "An Analysis of Cherokee Sorcery and Witchcraft." In *Four Centuries of Southern Indians*, edited by Charles M. Hudson, 113–31. Athens: University of Georgia Press, 1975.

———. "Who Were the Ani-Kutani? An Excursion into Cherokee Historical Thought." *Ethnohistory* 31 (Autumn 1984): 255–63.

Gallay, Alan. *The Indian Slave Trade: The Rise of the English Empire in the American South, 1670–1717*. New Haven, Conn.: Yale University Press, 2002.

Gearing, Fred. *Priests and Warriors: Social Structures for Cherokee Politics in the Eighteenth Century*. Menasha, Wisc.: American Anthropological Association, 1962.

Gibson, Jon L. "Aboriginal Warfare in the Protohistoric Southeast: An Alternative Perspective." *American Antiquity* 39 (January 1974): 130–33.

Goodwin, Gary C. *Cherokees in Transition: A Study of Changing Culture and Environment Prior to 1775*. Chicago: University of Chicago, 1977.

Griffin, James B. "Comments on Late Prehistoric Societies in the Southeast." In *Towns and Temples along the Mississippi*, edited by David H. Dye and Cheryl A. Cox, 5–15. Tuscaloosa: University of Alabama Press, 1990.

Haan, Richard L. "'The Trade Do's Not Flourish as Formerly': The Ecological Origins of the Yamasee War of 1715." *Ethnohistory* 28 (Fall 1981): 341–58.

Hahn, Steven C. *Invention of the Creek Nation, 1670–1763*. Lincoln: University of Nebraska Press, 2004.

Hally, David J. "Chiefdom of Coosa." In *The Forgotten Centuries: Indians and Europeans in the American South, 1521–1704*, edited by Charles Hudson and Carmen Chaves Tesser, 227–53. Athens: University of Georgia, 1994.

Halsey, Robert H. *How the President, Thomas Jefferson, and Doctor Benjamin Waterhouse Established Vaccination as a Public Health Procedure*. New York: published by the author, 1936.

Hann, John H. *Apalachee: The Land between the Rivers*. Gainesville: University Presses of Florida, 1988.

Harder, Ben. "The Seeds of Malaria: Recent Evolution Cultivated a Deadly Scourge." *Science News* 160 (November 10, 2001): 206–98.

Hatley, M. Thomas. *Dividing Paths: Cherokees and South Carolinians through the Era of Revolution*. New York: Oxford University Press, 1993.

———. "The Three Lives of Keowee: Loss and Recovery in the Eighteenth-Century Cherokee Villages." In *Powhatan's Mantle: Indians in the Colonial Southeast*, edited by Peter H. Wood, Gregory A. Walselkov, and M. Thomas Hatley, 223–48. Lincoln: University of Nebraska Press, 1989.

Haywood, John. *Natural and Aboriginal History of Tennessee: Up to the First Settlements therein by the White People, in the Year 1768*. Nashville: George Wilson, 1823.

———. *The Civil and Political History of the State of Tennessee from Its Earliest Settlement up to the Year, 1796*. Knoxville: Heiskell and Brown, 1823.

Henige, David. *Numbers from Nowhere: The American Indian Contact Population Debate*. Norman: University of Oklahoma, 1998.

Hewatt, Alexander. *An Historical Account of the Rise and Progress of the Colonies of South Carolina and Georgia*. 2 vols. London: A. Donaldson, 1779.

Hickerson, Harold. *The Southwestern Chippewa: An Ethnohistorical Study*. Menasha, Wisc.: George Banta Co., 1962.

Hoig, Stan. *The Cherokees and Their Chiefs: In the Wake of Empire*. Fayetteville: University of Arkansas Press, 1998.

Hudson, Charles. *Knights of Spain, Warriors of the Sun: Hernando de Soto and the South's Ancient Chiefdoms*. Athens: University of Georgia Press, 1997.

———. "Why the Southeastern Indians Slaughtered Deer." In *Indians, Animals, and the Fur Trade*, edited by Shepard Krech, 155–76.

Irwin, Lee. "Cherokee Healing: Myth, Dreams and Medicine." *American Indian Quarterly* 16 (Spring 1992): 237–57.

Ishii, Izumi. *Bad Fruits of the Civilized Tree: Alcohol and the Sovereignty of the Cherokee Nation*. Lincoln: University of Nebraska Press, 2008.

Jones, David S. "Death, Uncertainty, and Rhetoric." In *Beyond Germs*, edited by Cameron, et al.

———. *Rationalizing Epidemics: Meanings and Uses of American Indian Mortality since 1600*. Cambridge, Mass.: Harvard University Press, 2004.

———. "Virgin Soils Revisited." *William and Mary Quarterly* 60 (October 2003): 703–42.

Katz, Steven T. "The Uniqueness of the Holocaust: The Historical Dimension." In *Is the Holocaust Unique? Perspectives on Comparative Genocide*, edited by Alan S. Rosenbaum, 19–38. Boulder, Colo.: Westview Press, 1996.

Kelm, Mary Ellen. *Colonizing Bodies: Aboriginal Health and Healing in British Columbia, 1900–1950*. Vancouver: University of British Columbia Press, 1999.

Kelton, Paul. "Avoiding the Smallpox Spirits: Colonial Epidemics and Southeastern Indian Survival." *Ethnohistory* 51 (Winter 2004): 45–71.

———. "The British and Indian War: Cherokee Power and the Fate of Empire in North America." *William and Mary Quarterly* 69 (October 2012): 765–94.

———. *Epidemics and Enslavement: Biological Catastrophe in the Native Southeast*. Lincoln: University of Nebraska Press, 2007.

———. "The Great Southeastern Smallpox Epidemic." In *The Transformation of the Southeastern Indians*, edited by Robbie Ethridge and Charles Hudson, 21–37.

Kennedy, David, Lizabeth Cohen, and Thomas A. Bailey. *The American Pageant*. Boston: Houghton Mifflin Company, 2006.

Kilpatrick, Jack, and Anna G. Kilpatrick. *Friends of Thunder: Folktales of the Oklahoma Cherokees*. Dallas: Southern Methodist University Press, 1964.

———. *Run toward the Nightland: Magic of the Oklahoma Cherokees*. Dallas: Southern Methodist University Press, 1967.

———. *The Shadow of Sequoyah: Social Documents of the Cherokees, 1862–1964*. Norman: University of Oklahoma Press, 1965.

Kiple, Kenneth, ed. *Cambridge World History of Human Disease*. New York: Cambridge University Press, 1993.

Knollenberg, Bernhard. "General Amherst and Germ Warfare." *The Mississippi Valley Historical Review* 41 (December 1954): 489–94.

———. "Communications." *The Mississippi Valley Historical Review* 41 (March 1955): 762-63.

Krech, Shepard, ed. *Indians, Animals, and the Fur Trade: A Critique of Keepers of the Game*. Athens: University of Georgia Press, 1981.

———. *Spirits of the Air: Birds & American Indians in the South*. Athens: University of Georgia Press, 2009.

Kresbach, Suzanne. "The Great Charlestown Smallpox Epidemic of 1760." *South Carolina Historical Magazine* 97 (January 1996): 30–37.

Larson, Lewis H. "Functional Considerations of Warfare in the Southeast during the Mississippian Period." *American Antiquity* 37 (July 1972): 383–92.

La Vere, David. *The Tuscarora War: Indians, Settlers, and the Fight for the Carolina Colonies*. Chapel Hill: University of North Carolina Press, 2013.

LeBaron, Charles W., and David W. Taylor. "Typhoid Fever." In *Cambridge World History of Human Disease*, edited by Kenneth Kiple, 1071–77.

Livi Bacci, Massimo. *Conquest: The Destruction of the American Indios*. Translated by Carl Ipsen. Malden, Mass.: Polity Press, 2008.

Lumpkin, Henry. *From Savannah to Yorktown: The American Revolution in the South*. Columbia: University of South Carolina Press, 1981.

Lux, Maureen. *Medicine that Walks: Disease, Medicine, and Canadian Plains Native People, 1880–1940*. Toronto: University of Toronto Press, 2001.

MacGowen, D. J. "Indian Secret Societies." *Historical Magazine* 10 (1866): 139–41.

MacLeod, D. Peter. "Microbes and Muskets: Smallpox and the Participation of the Amerindian Allies of New France in the Seven Years' War." *Ethnohistory* 39 (Winter 1992): 42–64.

Mancall, Peter. *Deadly Medicine: Indians and Alcohol in Early America*. Ithaca, N.Y.: Cornell University Press, 1997.

Mann, Barbara Alice. *The Tainted Gift: The Disease Method of Frontier Expansion*. Denver, Colo.: Praeger, 2009.

Mann, Charles. *1491: New Revelations of the Americas before Columbus*. New York: Knopf, 2005.

Marble, Allan Everett. *Surgeons, Smallpox, and the Poor: A History of Medicine and Social Conditions in Nova Scotia, 1749–1799*. Montreal: McGill-Queen's University Press, 1997.

Martin, Calvin. *Keepers of the Game: Indian-Animal Relationships and the Fur Trade*. Berkeley: University of California Press, 1978.

Mayor, Adrienne. "The Nessus Shirt in the New World: Smallpox Blankets in History and Legend." *Journal of American Folklore* 108 (Winter 1995): 54–77.

McLoughlin, William. *Champions of the Cherokees: Evan and John B. Jones*. Princeton, N.J.: Princeton University Press, 1990.

———. *Cherokees and Missionaries, 1789–1839*. New Haven, Conn.: Yale University Press, 1984.

————. *Cherokee Renascence in the New Republic*. Princeton, N.J.: Princeton University Press, 1986.

McNeill, William. *Plagues and Peoples*. New York: Anchor Books, 1976.

Merbs, Charles F. "New World of Infectious Disease." *Yearbook of Physical Anthropology* 13 (1992): 3–42.

Merrell, James H. *The Indians' New World: Catawbas and Their Neighbors from European Contact through the Era of Removal*. New York: W. W. Norton, 1991.

Meyers, Maureen. "The Mississippian Frontier in Southwestern Virginia." *Southeastern Archaeology* 21 (Winter 2002): 178–91.

Miles, Tiya. *The House on Diamond Hill: A Cherokee Plantation Story*. Chapel Hill: University of North Carolina, 2010.

Milner, George. "Epidemic Disease in the Postcontact Southeast: A Reappraisal." *Mid-Continental Journal of Archaeology* 5 (1980): 39–56.

Milner, George R., David G. Anderson, and Marvin T. Smith. "The Distribution of Eastern Woodlands Peoples at the Prehistoric and Historic Interface." In *Societies in Eclipse: Archaeology of the Eastern Woodland Indians, A.D. 1400–1700*, edited by David S. Brose, C. Wesley Cowan, and Robert C. Mainfort, Jr., 9–18. Tuscaloosa: Universtiy of Alabama Press, 2001.

Mooney, James. *Aboriginal Population of America North of Mexico*. Washington, D.C.: Smithsonian Institution Press, 1928.

————. "The Cherokee River Cult." *Journal of American Folklore* 13 (January–March 1900): 1–10.

_____. *The Sacred Formulas of the Cherokees*. In *Seventh Annual Report of the Bureau of Ethnology, 1885–86*. Washington, D.C.: Government Printing Office, 1891.

————. *History, Myths, and Sacred Formulas of the Cherokees*. Asheville, N.C.: Historical Images, 1992.

Moore, David G. *Catawba Valley Mississippian: Ceramics, Chronology, and Catawba Indians*. Tuscaloosa: University of Alabama Press, 2002.

Morgan, Edmund S. *American Slavery/American Freedom: The Ordeal of Colonial Virginia*. New York: W. W. Norton, 1975.

Moulton, Gary. *John Ross, Cherokee Chief*. Athens: University of Georgia Press, 1978.

Muller, Jon. *Mississippian Political Economy*. New York: Plenum Press, 1997.

Oatis, Steven J. *A Colonial Complex: South Carolina's Frontiers in the Era of the Yamasee War, 1680–1730*. Lincoln: University of Nebraska Press, 2004.

O'Donnell, James, III. *Southern Indians in the American Revolution*. Knoxville: University of Tennessee Press, 1973.

Olbrechts, Frans M., ed. *The Swimmer Manuscript: Cherokee Sacred Formulas and Medicinal Prescriptions*. Washington, D.C.: U.S. Government Printing Office, 1932.

Oliphant, John. *Peace and War on the Anglo-Cherokee Frontier, 1756–63*. Baton Rouge: Louisiana State University Press, 2001.

Parkman, Francis. *The Conspiracy of Pontiac and the Indian War after the Conquest of Canada*. 3 vols. 9th ed. Boston: Little, Brown, 1899.

Pauketat, Timothy R. *The Ascent of Chiefs*. Tuscaloosa: University of Alabama Press, 1994.

Pauketat, Timothy R., and Thomas E. Emerson, eds. *Cahokia: Domination and Ideology in the Mississippian World*. Lincoln: University of Nebraska Press, 1997.

Pearson, J. Diane. "Medical Diplomacy and the American Indian: Thomas Jefferson, the Lewis and Clark Expedition, and the Subsequent Effects on American Indian Health and Public Policy." *Wicazo Sa Review* 19 (Spring 2004): 105–30.

Peebles, Christopher S., and Susan M. Kus. "Some Archaeological Correlates of Ranked Societies." *American Antiquity* 42 (July 1977): 421–48.

Perdue, Theda. "Cherokee Relations with the Iroquois." In *Beyond the Covenant Chain: The Iroquois and Their Neighbors in Indian North America, 1600–1800*, edited by Daniel K. Richter and James H. Merrell, 135–49. Syracuse: Syracuse University Press, 1987.

———. *Cherokee Women: Gender and Culture Change, 1700–1835*. Lincoln: University of Nebraska Press, 1998.

———. *Slavery and the Evolution of Cherokee Society, 1540–1866*. Knoxville: University of Tennessee Press, 1979.

Perdue, Theda, and Michael D. Green. *The Cherokee Nation and the Trail of Tears*. New York: Viking, 2007.

Piecuch, Jim. *Three Peoples, One King: Loyalists, Indians, and Slaves in the Revolutionary South, 1775–1782*. Columbia: University of South Carolina Press, 2008.

Putnam, A. W. *History of Middle Tennessee: or, Life and Times of General James Robertson*. Nashville: printed for the author, 1859.

Ramenofsky, Ann. "Diseases of the Americas, 1492–1700." In *Cambridge World History of Human Disease*, edited by Kenneth Kiple, 323.

———. *Vectors of Death: The Archaeology of European Contact*. Albuquerque: University of New Mexico Press, 1987.

Ramenofsky, Ann F., and Patricia Galloway. "Disease and the Soto Entrada." In *The Hernando de Soto Expedition: History, Historiography, and "Discovery" in the Southeast*, edited by Patricia Galloway, 259–80. Lincoln: University of Nebraska Press, 2005.

Ramsey, James G. M. *The Annals of Tennessee to the End of the Eighteenth Century*. Charleston, S.C.: Walker and James, 1853. Reprint, Kingsport, Tenn.: Kingsport Press, 1926.

Ramsey, William L. "'Something Cloudy in Their Looks': The Origins of the Yamasee War Reconsidered." *Journal of American History* 90 (June 2003): 44–75.

Reff, Daniel. *Disease, Depopulation, and Culture Change in Northwestern New Spain*. Salt Lake City: University of Utah Press, 1991.

Reid, John Philip. *A Better Kind of Hatchet: Law, Trade, and Diplomacy in the Cherokee Nation during the Early Years of European Contact*. University Park: Pennsylvania State University Press, 1976.

Richter, Daniel K. *Ordeal of the Longhouse: The Peoples of the Iroquois League in the Era of European Colonization*. Chapel Hill: University of North Carolina Press, 1992.

Riley, James. "Smallpox and American Indians Revisited." *Journal of the History of Medicine and Allied Sciences* 65 (October 2010): 445–77.

Roberts, Wayne D. "Lithic Artifacts." In *The Toqua Site: A Late Mississippian Dallas Phase Town*, edited by Richard R. Polhemus, 689–909. University of Tennessee

Department of Anthropology, Report of Investigations 41, Tennessee Valley Authority Publications in Anthropology, 44. Knoxville: Tennessee Valley Authority, 1987.

Roosevelt, Theodore. *The Winning of the West*. 4 vols. New York: G. P. Putnam's Sons, 1889.

Schlesier, Karl H. "Epidemics and Indian Middlemen: Rethinking the Wars of the Iroquois, 1609–1653." *Ethnohistory* 23 (Spring 1976): 129–45.

Schmidt, Ethan. *The Divided Dominion: Social Conflict and Indian Hatred in Early Virginia*. Boulder: University Press of Colorado, 2014.

————. *Native Americans in the American Revolution: How the War Divided, Devastated, and Transformed the Early American Indian World*. Santa Barbara, Calif.: Praeger, 2014.

Sheehan, Bernard W. *Seeds of Extinction: Jeffersonian Philanthropy and the American Indian*. Chapel Hill: University of North Carolina Press, 1973.

Shurkin, Joel N. *Invisible Fire: The Story of Mankind's Victory over the Ancient Scourge of Smallpox*. New York: Putnam, 1979.

Smith, Marvin T. *Archaeology of Aboriginal Culture Change in the Interior Southeast: Depopulation during the Early Historic Period*. Gainesville: University Press of Florida, 1987.

————. *Coosa: The Rise and Fall of a Southeastern Mississippian Chiefdom*. Gainesville: University Press of Florida, 2000.

Snow, Dean, and Kim M. Lanphear, "European Contact and Indian Depopulation in the Northeast: The Timing of the First Epidemics." *Ethnohistory* 35 (Winter 1988): 15–33.

Stearn, E. Wagner, and Allen E. Stearn. *The Effect of Smallpox on the Destiny of the Amerindian*. Boston: Bruce Humphries, 1945.

Steinen, Karl T. "Ambushes, Raids, and Palisades: Mississippian Warfare in the Interior Southeast." *Southeastern Archaeology* 11 (Winter 1992): 132–39.

Steponaitis, Vincas. "Contrasting Patterns of Mississippian Development." In *Chiefdoms: Power, Economy, and Ideology*, ed. Timothy Earle, 193–228. New York: Cambridge University Press, 1997.

Stevens, William B. *A History of Georgia, from Its First Discovery by Europeans to the Adoption of the Present Constitution in 1798*. Vol. 2. Philadelphia: E. H. Butler, 1859.

Swanton, John. *Early History of the Creek Indians and Their Neighbors*. Washington, D.C.: Government Printing Office, 1922.

Thornton, Russell. *The Cherokees: A Population History*. Lincoln: University of Nebraska Press, 1990.

Townsend, Richard F. *The Aztecs*. 2nd ed. London: Thames and Hudson, 2000.

Valenčius, Conevery Bolton. *The Health of the Country: How American Settlers Understood Themselves and Their Land*. New York: Basic Books, 2002.

Wallace, Anthony F. C. *Jefferson and the Indians: The Tragic Fate of the First Americans*. Cambridge, Mass.: Harvard University Press, 1999.

Ward, H. Trawick, and R. P. Stephen Davis, Jr. *Time before History: The Archaeology of North Carolina*. Chapel Hill: University of North Carolina Press, 1999.

Ward, Matthew. *Breaking the Backcountry: The Seven Years' War in Virginia and Pennsylvania, 1754–1765*. Pittsburgh, Pa.: University of Pittsburgh Press, 2003.

———. "The Microbes of War: The British Army and the Ohio Indians, 1758–1774." In *The Sixty Years War for the Great Lakes*, edited by David K. Skaggs and Larry L. Nelson, 63–78. East Lansing: Michigan State University Press, 2001.

Warrick, Gary. "European Infectious Disease and Depopulation of the Wendat-Tionontate (Huron-Petun)." *World Archaeology* 35 (2003): 258–75.

Waselkov, Gregory A. "The Macon Trading House and Early European-Indian Contact in the Colonial Southeast." In *Ocmulgee Archaeology, 1936-1986*, edited by David J. Hally, 190–96. Athens: University of Georgia Press, 1994.

———. "Seventeenth-Century Trade in the Colonial Southeast." *Southeastern Archaeology* 8 (Winter 1989): 117–33.

Watts, Sheldon. *Epidemics and History: Disease, Power and Imperialism*. New Haven, Conn.: Yale University Press, 1997.

Welch, Paul D. *Moundville's Economy*. Tuscaloosa: University of Alabama Press, 1991.

Widmer, Randolph J. "The Structure of Southeastern Chiefdoms." In *The Forgotten Centuries: Indians and Europeans in the American South, 1521–1704*, edited by Charles Hudson and Carmen Chaves Tesser, 125–55. Athens: University of Georgia, 1994.

Wood, Peter. "The Changing Population of the Colonial South: An Overview by Race and Region." In *Powhatan's Mantle: Indians in the Colonial Southeast*, edited by Peter H. Wood, Gregory A. Walselkov, and M. Thomas Hatley, 35–103. Lincoln: University of Nebraska Press, 1989.

———. "The Impact of Smallpox on the Native Population of the 18th-century South." *New York State Journal of Medicine* 87 (January 1987): 30–36.

Worth, John E. *The Timucuan Chiefdoms of Spanish Florida*. 2 vols. Gainesville: University Press of Florida, 1998.

Zinsser, Hans. *Rats, Lice, and History*. Boston: Little, Brown, 1935.

Zogry, Michael J. *Anetso, the Cherokee Ball Game: At the Center of Ceremony and Identity*. Chapel Hill: University of North Carolina Press, 2010.

INDEX

Page numbers in *italics* indicate illustrations.